Vaccines

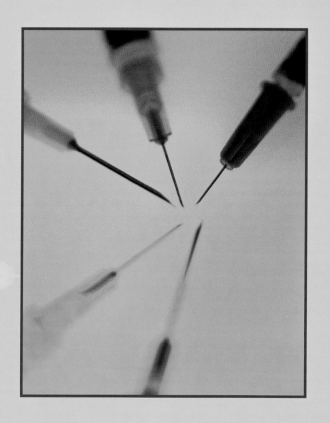

GREAT INVENTIONS

Vaccines

JAMES LINCOLN COLLIER

BENCHMARK BOOKS

MARSHALL CAVENDISH
NEW YORK

⌐═━⊷

Benchmark Books
Marshall Cavendish
99 White Plains Road
Tarrytown, NY 10591-9001
www.marshallcavendish.com
Text copyright © 2004 by James Lincoln Collier

All Internet sites were available and accurate when sent to press.

Library of Congress Cataloging-in-Publication Data

Collier, James Lincoln, 1928–
Vaccines / James Lincoln Collier.
p. cm.—(Great inventions)
Summary: Explains the diseases that led to the discovery of vaccines, how vaccines work, and how that has changed the history of medicine.
Includes bibliographical references and index.
ISBN 0-7614-1539-4
1. Vaccines—Juvenile literature. [1. Vaccines.] I. Title.
II. Series: Great inventions (Benchmark Books (Firm))

RM281.C645 2003
615'.372—dc21   2002156287

Photo research by James Lincoln Collier

Series design by Sonia Chaghatzbanian

Cover photo: Corbis

The photographs in this book are used by permission and through the courtesy of:
Corbis: 2, 39, 40-41, 57; Historical Picture Archive, 12-13, 52-53; Christie's Images, 24, 116-117; Bettmann, 35, 36-37, 44, 60, 73, 79, 88; Nicole Duplaix, 47; Bojan Brecelj, 74; Hulton-Deutsch Collection, 80; AFP, 85, 115; Ed Bock, 86; Peter Turnley, 104; Reuters New Media Inc., 108, 111, 112-113. New York Public Library: 8, 14-15, 17, 20, 28, 50, 54, 64, 68, 76. Museum of the City of New York: 67. March of Dimes Birth Defects Foundation: 91, 93, 94, 98, 101.

Printed in China

1 3 5 6 4 2

CONTENTS

One   "And No Bells Tolled"   9

Two   Doctor Jenner's Milkhands   25

Three   Death Invisible   45

Four   Cleaning up the Cities   65

Five   The Forgotten Plague   77

Six   The Great Crippler   89

Seven   The Future   105

Web Sites   119

Bibliography   121

Index   123

Vaccines

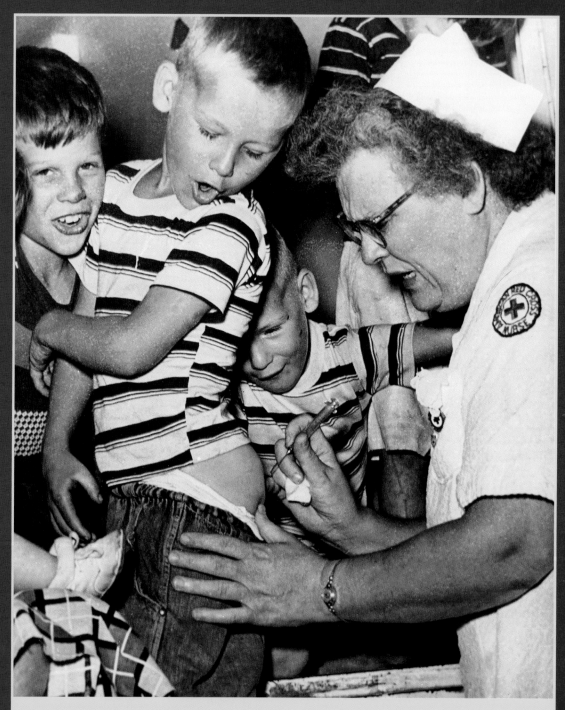

After a 1951 flood in St. Louis, Missouri, these boys were given typhoid shots. To them it was a small matter, but in the recent past typhoid fever was a deadly disease that killed tens of thousands of people annually.

ONE

"And No Bells Tolled"

Over the millennia, and particularly over the past several hundred years, people have invented countless instruments and systems for doing things that have vastly improved human life. These range from the earliest bronze axes to the most recent computers, from dugout canoes to supersonic jets. Probably none of these things has so profoundly aided humanity as the invention of vaccines. For those of us living in the industrial world with the benefits of modern medicine easily available to us, it is almost impossible to imagine how different life was for most people even 200 years ago. Then most infectious diseases could not be cured, much less prevented.

It was a time when everybody, both princes and paupers, lived with the knowledge that they could, at any moment, be struck by a deadly disease that seemed to come out of nowhere, but that might kill them in a matter of hours. It was a time when, from childhood, death was a constant presence, when few people reached their teen years without having lost somebody close to them—a parent, a brother, or a sister. It was a time when fathers and mothers took it for granted that at least one, and perhaps two or three, of their children would die young. England's Queen Anne, who reigned 300 years ago, had seventeen children, all of whom died very young. When Queen Anne died, the English had to search out a distant German relative of Anne's to be their new king. He didn't even speak English. Still he established the royal line from which the present English monarch descended.

If you did not die in childhood, you might not live very long either: it was usual for people to die in their thirties and forties. Men or women in their fifties were thought to be old, and somebody who lived to be seventy was remarkable. And it was a time when, no matter where in the world you lived, a scourge might suddenly appear that would sweep away whole families, whole streets of people, half a town, or a third of a nation. To understand how devastating disease could be in a time before modern medicine, we will look at a moment in history when it appeared that an angry god had indeed decided to terminate life on Earth.

Roughly before the year A.D. 1000, Europe—especially the northwestern part of Europe—was a minor backwater, with nothing like the arts and sciences that existed in China or the Muslim world. Technology was at a standstill. European civilization had gone backward since the great days of the Roman Empire a thousand years before, when paved roads ran for hundreds of miles between walled cities surrounded by elegant villas with marbled floors, pools, and frescoed walls. By A.D. 1000 the villas had been torn down to make cowsheds, and the roads were overgrown.

Then, in the years between A.D. 900 and A.D. 1300, things began to change. Improvements in agriculture, especially the introduction of a better plow, allowed more land to be cleared and planted. Several centuries of milder weather helped, and during this period, Europe suffered from few serious epidemics. People's health improved. The population grew and grew again, doubling over these centuries. Some of these new people pushed eastward into the sparsely settled land around what is now Poland. But many of them were forced from farms into towns. Villages grew into towns, towns into cities. The swelling population needed jobs, and soon enterprising city dwellers set up small but growing industries in textiles, glassmaking, and metalworking.

Once again there were technological improvements, and factory output increased. Trade sprang up among these burgeoning cities, especially seaports such as Venice and Genoa, and then spread across the Mediterranean into North Africa and the Middle East. There was money to be made in trade, and the lure of wealth drove technology further ahead. Better ways of making paper, steel, glass, and cloth were devised. Ships capable of sailing longer distances were built. Navigational instruments were improved, and around 1290 the first practical clocks were built.

By 1300 Europeans were beginning to establish great traditions in the areas of painting, sculpture, literature, and music. Universities were founded, first in Paris and then everywhere.

Then the period of mild weather ended, and what historians call the Little Ice Age began, lasting into the nineteenth century. This change in the weather was not immediately discernible, but another disaster was. Sometime in the 1340s in Central Asia, a deadly disease broke out. It spread rapidly into China and India, and in 1346 reached the Crimea, along the Black Sea, where the Italian city of Genoa had a colony. The colony was being besieged by Tatar warriors. Historians believe the Tatars catapulted the bodies of plague victims into the colony. The defenders leaped into boats and fled back to Europe. They stopped first at Messina, in Sicily. By this time a few of the sailors in the galleys were sick with an ugly disease. Deep black swellings the size of an egg festered in their armpits and groins, from which oozed blood and pus. Other victims coughed and spit blood. All suffered intense agony and nearly all died within eight days, many within three.

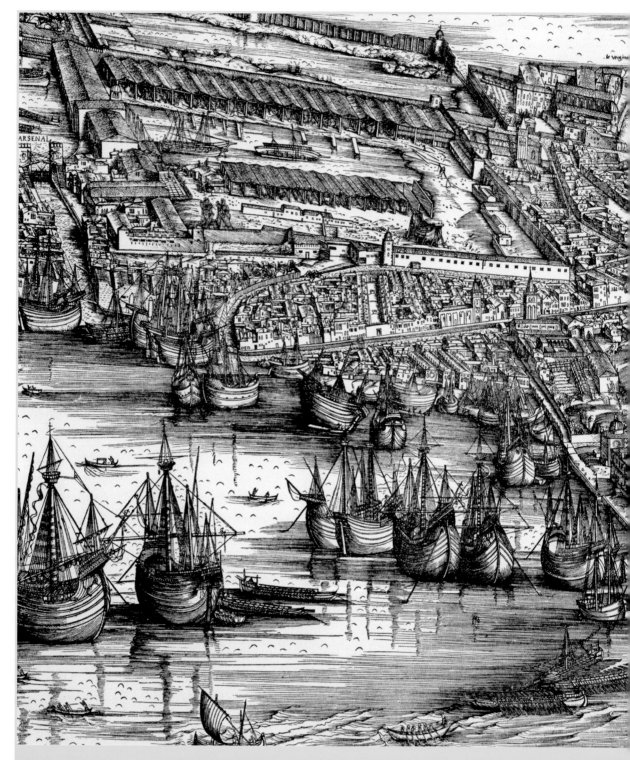

EUROPE'S ADVANCES IN TECHNOLOGY WERE BROUGHT ABOUT IN PART BY THE SUDDEN INCREASE IN TRADE.
PORT CITIES SUCH AS VENICE WITH ITS NATURAL, WELL-PROTECTED HARBOR EMERGED AS MAJOR ECONOMIC

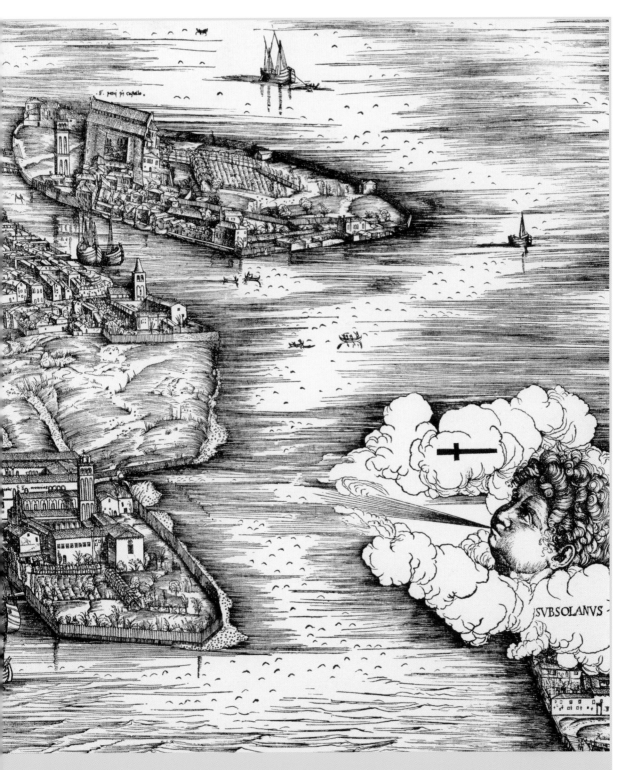

CENTERS. THE GROWING COMMERCE BROUGHT PROSPERITY, BUT IT ALSO BROUGHT MICROBES FROM NEAR AND FAR. THEY OFTEN SPREAD RAPIDLY THROUGH THE COUNTRYSIDE, TRIGGERING PLAGUES.

This was bubonic plague. (There is some confusion about the word *plague*: sometimes it means bubonic plague specifically; at other times it covers any kind of serious epidemic.) Today this particular epidemic is referred to as the Black Death, but at the time was called the pestilence, or simply the pest. Whatever the name, it spread quickly. It moved especially fast along the European coast, carried by the very ships that were making European traders wealthy. But it moved inland too, spreading north from Italy through France and Switzerland into Germany, the Netherlands, England, and Scandinavia. Through 1348 and 1349 it prevailed, until its deadly hand touched everywhere—not only Europe, but Asia and elsewhere as well. In the smaller towns it often died out in the winter, but in the big cities such as Paris and Venice that had populations of around 100,000, it might lay dormant in winter only to flare up again in the spring, bringing another round of death to besiege the residents who had thought they had escaped it.

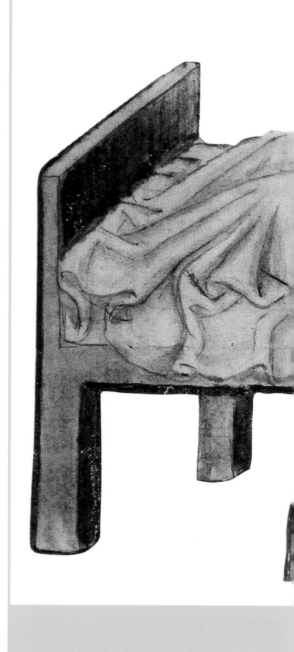

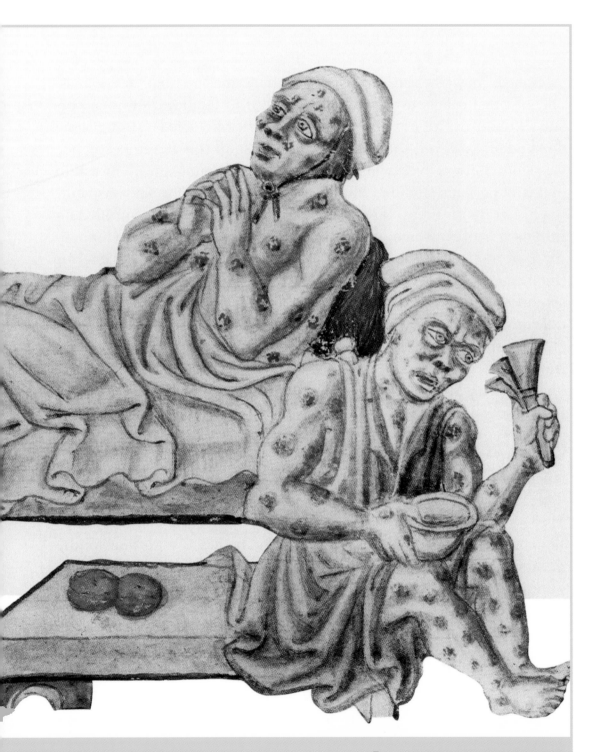

BUBONIC PLAGUE WAS AS UNATTRACTIVE AS IT WAS PAINFUL. FESTERING SPOTS ERUPTED ON THE BODY. PEOPLE WHO SAW THESE TELLTALE SIGNS EMERGE ON THEIR SKIN KNEW THAT THEY WERE PROBABLY DOOMED TO DIE.

Nobody knew the cause. Did it come from some "miasma," some invisible mist that caught everyone it touched? Did it jump from one person's breath to the next, as some authorities believed? Most people concluded, however, that the ultimate cause of this fierce pestilence was God. Sin was everywhere, that was clear; humans were awash in evil, and perhaps God had finally sickened at the sight and was venting his wrath on them. Indeed, as the assault of the disease rolled on into its third year, some concluded that God intended to wipe humanity from the face of the earth. They had good reason to believe it, for the plague was ferocious. It hit particularly hard the monks and nuns sequestered in monasteries and convents—people who lived in close quarters. There, when the plague struck, the residents often died so fast that the living could not keep up with the burials, but stayed surrounded by the corpses of their fellows. In some monasteries everyone perished. Matters were not much better outside monastery walls. In many villages the locals had to be buried in mass graves. In horror, people watched their families and friends fall and die, until the few who were left alive crept away and the village fell into ruins, the roofs fallen in, grass growing in the streets.

It was just as bad in the cities. In Paris 50,000 people died—at least a third and perhaps half of the population. In Venice the death rate was similar, in Florence one-half. Everywhere bodies lay rotting in the streets. In Avignon, France, when the graveyards were full, the bodies were thrown in the Rhône River to rot and stink. In London the dead were heaved into great pits. In some places family members were required to bury their own husbands, wives, or children. Nobody else would touch the bodies. Fearful of catching the disease, the relatives dug hastily, sometimes covering up the bodies with only a few inches of dirt. There was a horror in the plague that went beyond the fear of death; the bubonic plague was hideous to look at, and it stank. At its approach people fled. Parents left sickened children, and wives left husbands to die alone in their agony. Some priests refused to offer victims the last rites.

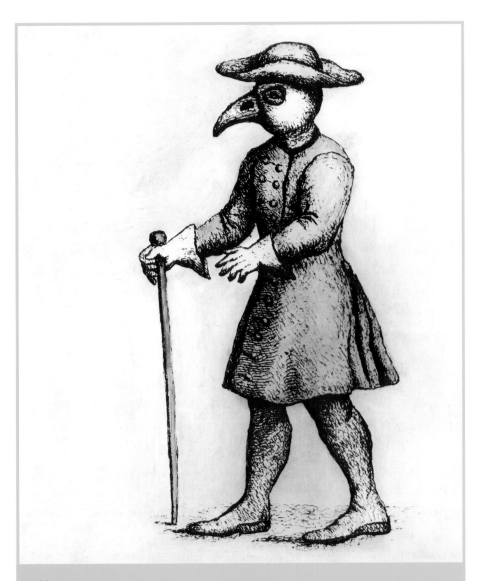

Medieval doctors sometimes wore protective masks, along with gloves and leg coverings, to help ward off disease. The beak of the mask was filled with herbs and spices, which were supposed to counteract the disease, which many thought hung invisibly in the air around them.

Often doctors would not come, as there was little they could do to ease a patient.

People, facing what seemed to be certain death, abandoned all pretense of morality. A dark despair pervaded. Morale was low, and some people lost all concern for others. "And no bells tolled," wrote one witness, "and nobody wept no matter what his loss because almost everyone expected death. . . ."

Inevitably people looked around for somebody to blame, and their eyes fell upon the Jews. Religious freedom did not exist in fourteenth-century Europe. The Roman Catholic Church was the only accepted religion, and in most cases kings and queens required their subjects to belong to it, usually under threat of execution.

An exception was made for Jews, who were allowed to worship in their traditional manner. Nonetheless their customs seemed strange, and there was always an undercurrent of dislike for Jews among many Christians.

As the Black Death claimed more lives, the rumor spread that it had been caused by Jews. The story was passed around that Jews had been sent from somewhere—the place varied—to dump poison into the wells of Christians. In some towns Jews were pulled from their homes by the hundreds and flung onto fires. In other places they were herded into houses especially built for the purpose, and then the houses were set on fire. In Strasbourg some 2,000 Jews were taken out to a burial ground, and all those who would not convert to Christianity were burned at the stake.

Not everybody believed the well-poisoning story, though, and there were cases where town authorities tried to prevent the massacre of Jews. Pope Clement attempted to halt the killings. In a papal edict he pointed out that Jews were dying from the plague along with everybody else, and ordered his clergy to protect them. But nobody paid any attention. By this time reason had long since departed.

Another reaction to the Black Death was an even greater focus on religion. This religious flame was curious, for many Europeans were behaving in a distinctly unchristian way, with their debauchery, slaughter of the Jews, and abandonment of sick friends and family. But these religious enthusiasts believed that they—and possibly the entire human race—were doomed, so they clutched desperately at the consolations of religion.

People thought that if they did penance for their sins, and the sins of humankind, God might be merciful. Groups of men and women appeared in the streets stripped to their waists, lashing their own backs with whips, often until they bled. Very quickly their numbers increased, until parades of penitents, as they were called, were a common sight in the streets of European cities. They were watched avidly by the local populations, who thought that possibly God would listen to the cries of the penitentials and lift the deadly scourge that afflicted everyone. The penitents were seen as potential saviors, admired and celebrated. Inevitably they became arrogant. Their leaders began to take on the authority of priests. Often mobs of penitents surged into Jewish quarters and massacred people. Finally it appeared that the penitents were about to incite rebellion and threaten both church and state. The rebellion had gone too far and was condemned by the pope. Secular rulers issued laws forbidding public whipping and executed some of the movement's leaders. The penitential movement quickly lost its popularity.

By 1350 the plague was dying out, although there would be sporadic outbreaks for hundreds of years: Vienna in 1576, London in 1665, Marseilles in 1721. A third of the population of Europe, perhaps 20 million people, had died. And still nobody knew what had caused the pestilence, why it had come upon them so swiftly, why it killed so ruthlessly, and why it had disappeared as silently as it had come. It was not until fairly recently that scientists and historians cleared up the mystery of the Black Death. We now know that it came in two forms, transmitted in different ways. The main strain of the bubonic plague was carried by

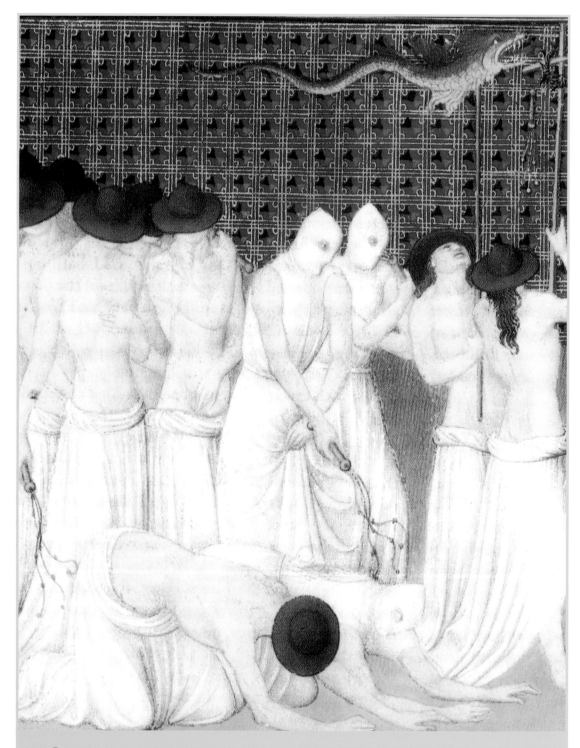

PENITENTS PARADED THROUGH CITIES IN THE HOPES THAT IF THEY PUNISHED THEMSELVES FOR
THEIR SINS THEIR LIVES WOULD BE SPARED. THESE PENITENTS ARE CARRYING A CROSS TO WHICH A
DRAGON-FISH EMBLEM, A SYMBOL OF THE DEVIL, WAS ATTACHED. THE FISH REPRESENTED CHRIST
CAPTURING AND DEFEATING THE DEVIL.

a certain species of rat that could pass on the disease by biting a human. The plague was also transmitted by the bites of fleas that lived on the rats.

The rats were good climbers and could easily make their way up the heavy lines used to tie ships to their docks. These ships were often carrying grain, fruit, and other foodstuffs that attracted the rats. They climbed onto the ships, which sailed off with the rats still onboard. In this way the Black Death was carried from Asia to Europe where it spread with devastating speed. Another strain of the disease was spread by droplets of moisture in the breath of the infected. People who feared to tend to their own sick were right in believing that they might catch the disease from them.

The effects of the plague on European society were diffuse, but they were real and they were far reaching. Before the Black Death, Europe had seen a substantial increase in population, and there were too many people looking for jobs. After the plague this excess ended, and a shortage of labor occurred. Workers were now less easy to intimidate because they could always find another employer. They forced wages up and demanded better working conditions. Laborers were still a long way from getting a fair share of the results of their toil, but they had taken strides toward improving their lives.

The Black Death also signaled the end of the old feudal system. That is a complex subject, which historians continue to debate. Put simply, feudalism was a system under which a small aristocracy, which controlled most of the land, kept a majority of the people in a form of semislavery. The labor shortage produced by the Black Death, by increasing somewhat the power of serfs, helped to push Europe toward an economy in which money, not land, was the source of power. Over time, traders, shippers, and factory owners began to assume power at the expense of the hereditary dukes and counts who had formerly ruled with absolute authority. Although the money-based economy had already been established before 1347, the Black Death hastened it along.

In our look at vaccines, there is an important lesson to be learned from the story of the Black Death. It was not the first horrifying event of its kind, but one of a great many epidemics, large and small, that had scourged humanity. One historian has found records of almost three hundred epidemics in China alone between 243 B.C. and A.D. 1911. That works out to about one every seven years. For some, epidemics were simply a way of life.

The effects of the major epidemics have often had a great impact on history. In 430 B.C., when the city-state of Athens was at the height of its golden age, an epidemic swept through the area. It lasted for more than two years and killed a third of the population.

One writer has said that the victims' "bodies broke out in sores that became ulcers; sleepless and agitated, unable to bear the touch of clothes or bedding, they staggered naked through the streets, seeking water for their unquenchable thirst." What, precisely, the disease was, historians are not sure. But Athens, which in this period had produced some of the world's greatest artists, writers, sculptors, and philosophers, rapidly declined. Had it not been for this epidemic, there is no telling what further glories Athens might have achieved. But there were other plagues to come.

Epidemics weakened civilizations, but above all, they affected the lives of individuals. Think how it must have been for people to see their friends and family taken in a matter of days, to live knowing that death was loitering around the corner. For years after the Black Death, the art of the 1300s was awash in images of death—skeletons and hooded figures bearing scythes. During times of epidemic there was no escape from the stink of rotting corpses in the streets, from a city turned into a death camp.

But in discussing vaccines, we need to look beyond epidemics. Even when a disease was not at an epidemic stage, it could remain a minor presence in a population. Smallpox, for example, was always claiming some victims, even when it was not responsible for the deaths of large numbers of people. Thus, before the era of modern medicine, there were always people showing symptoms of bubonic plague, smallpox, cholera, and many, many more infections that, even if the infections did not kill them, could leave them disfigured or blind. Before recent times, serious illness was routine, a regular part of human life every-where.

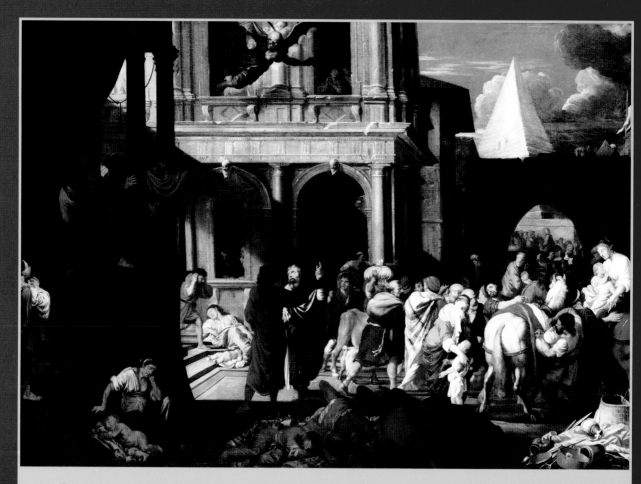

THE FEAR OF PLAGUES PREOCCUPIED PEOPLE FOR CENTURIES. THIS SEVENTEENTH-CENTURY PAINTING SHOWS A ROMAN CITY IN THE GRIP OF A PLAGUE. THE DEAD AND DYING LITTER THE STREETS, WHILE THE ANGEL OF DEATH HOVERS OVERHEAD.

Doctor Jenner's Milkhands

The bubonic plague is one of many hundreds of infectious diseases that have brought suffering, terror, and death to human beings over our long history. However, not all illnesses are caused by infection. Some are due to injury—an ankle twisted while skateboarding, a cut from a carelessly handled fishing knife, a rib cracked in a fall from a ladder. Other illnesses are caused by the lack of an essential vitamin. The most famous example is scurvy, a lack of vitamin C that used to be common in sailors who went without fresh fruit and vegetables for long periods at sea. Scurvy was prevented when it was discovered that if the sailors were regularly given limes—a source of vitamin C—they never got the disease, although at the time nobody knew why limes worked. Other diseases are caused by environmental factors—cancer brought on by exposure to cigarette smoke or respiratory illnesses provoked by smog and automobile exhausts. Still others are due to the malfunction of genes. Among these are autoimmune diseases such as multiple sclerosis, which can occur when the immune system attacks some part of the body.

So people can be made ill by a lot of things, but without a doubt we are far more frequently beset by infectious diseases than by any other type of illness. They have killed more people than all the wars and accidents humans have suffered. Just to cite one example, the almost forgotten influenza epidemic of 1918—which we will later examine—killed at least four times more people in a tenth of the time than the famous World War I that was going on simultaneously.

Bubonic plague has caused terrible suffering to human beings for millennia. One researcher has called the fourteenth-century plague "the worst disaster in human history." Yet over the course of human history at least one other disease has killed more people than either influenza or the plague—smallpox. There have been many smallpox epidemics, but the disease has always been endemic as well, striking a person here, another there in a regular way year after year, only to break out in an epidemic for a while, possibly several years, and then die down again, like a smoldering fire that occasionally flares up.

There are two primary types of smallpox, *variola major* and *variola minor*. The more powerful version killed 10 to 20 percent of its victims, the minor version only 1 percent. The disease began with a two-week incubation period, during which it gathered strength in the victim's body. Then came a very high fever, powerful headaches and backaches, and nausea. Ugly pus-filled boils appeared on the skin of the face and other parts of the body. The victim was tormented by thirst, but the throat infection made it too painful for him or her to swallow water. For days the victims lay in agony, then they either died or slowly began to improve.

But the agony did not end with the disease. As the pustules receded, they left deep pits in the skin, viciously scarring the faces of the sufferers. Until fairly recently the scarred faces of smallpox victims were a common sight in every nation in the world. Many victims were left partially or wholly blind. And of course they were the ones who survived. As late as the 1960s, some 10 to 15 million people got smallpox each year, and 2 million of them died in agony.

Given the death toll, it is hardly surprising that smallpox has had profound effects on human history. Although it is difficult to be sure about ancient illnesses, historians tend to think that the plague that helped to bring down the great Roman Empire was smallpox. One theory is that the disease was brought to Europe from Asia by conquering Huns, a fierce nomadic people who at one time struck terror into their neighbors. Whatever the case, by A.D. 164 the Roman Empire, although facing many troubles, was still the most powerful force in the world. Around A.D. 165, Roman soldiers who had been fighting in the Middle East brought smallpox back to Rome with them. For the next fifteen years it surfaced again and again in various places. A quarter to a third of the population of Italy died in those years; in Europe as a whole the death toll was 4 to 7 million people. A hundred years later, in the years A.D. 251 to 266, a second plague hit, once again probably smallpox. The death rate was enormous: at its peak the epidemic killed 5,000 people a day in the city of Rome alone. People fled to the countryside, but the disease followed them and went on killing.

These two smallpox plagues were by no means alone in destroying the once-mighty Roman Empire, but they were a major factor. The armed forces of an empire of that size needs millions of soldiers, sailors, and arms makers, who have to be fed. The sharply reduced Roman population left fewer farmers available to produce the extra food needed to support the troops guarding the frontiers. Year after year the empire receded, until enemies poured in and finished it off. More recently smallpox was a major factor in destroying the culture of the people native to what we now call the Americas. By the time of Columbus, there may have been as many as 70 million Indians living from what is now Canada down to the tip of South America. They lived in various ways: hunting and gathering, growing corn, or hunting sea creatures such as seals and whales. Some of these people, such as the Aztecs of Mexico and the Incas of Peru, had built civilizations with cities, temples, and great stores of gold and silver.

These people had been isolated from Europe for at least 10,000

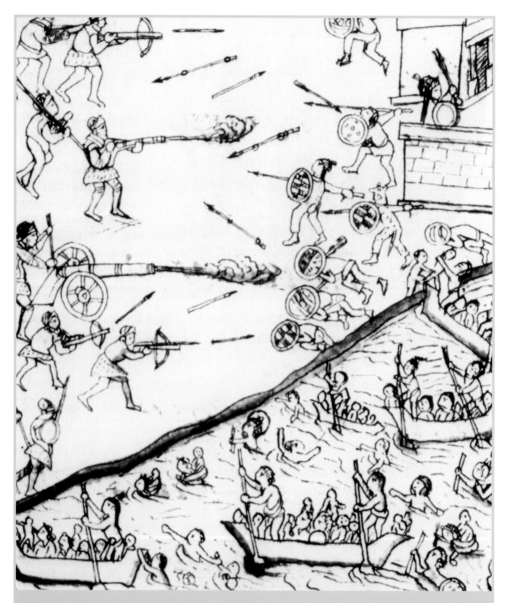

SPANISH CONQUISTADORS ARMED WITH CROSSBOWS, GUNS, AND CANNONS FIGHT SPEAR-
WIELDING AZTECS IN THE BATTLE FOR THE AZTEC CAPITAL OF TENOCHTITLÁN. WHILE THE
MORE LETHAL WEAPONS OF THE EUROPEANS HELPED THEM CONQUER MANY OF THE PEOPLES
OF THE AMERICAS, EUROPEAN DISEASES, TO WHICH THE INDIANS HAD NO NATURAL IMMUNITY,
WERE A CRITICAL FACTOR AS WELL. SMALLPOX ALONE KILLED FAR MORE INDIANS THAN
EUROPEAN GUNS.

years and probably much longer. They had not developed any resistance to the diseases that were common in the Old World. Europeans were by no means totally immune to smallpox and other infectious diseases, but they had developed a considerable resistance to them. Probably fewer than a quarter of those Europeans infected with smallpox died, and once they had recovered from the disease they could never get it again. But in a population that had never been exposed to the disease, the death rate could be enormous. That was the case in the New World.

Smallpox was not the only European disease to affect the Indians: measles, bubonic plague, and others swept through Indian villages and towns. But smallpox was the leader. Perhaps the best-known outbreak occurred when the Spaniard Hernán Cortés with a handful of soldiers came to Mexico determined to conquer it. They had with them an African slave who had a mild case of smallpox. Like Europeans, Africans were used to the disease. From this single source, smallpox swept through the Aztec capital of Tenochtitlán, until the city's canals were filled with corpses. Cortés later said, "A man could not set his foot down unless on the corpse of an Indian." Not only did smallpox compromise the Aztecs' ability to fight, it broke their morale: obviously the Spaniards' God was more powerful than the Aztecs'. Why else would Mexicans die of a disease that left the Spanish untouched? Soon the Spanish ruled Mexico, enslaving its people and stripping it of its wealth. Using the wealth it had seized from its New World colonies, Spain became the most powerful nation in Europe.

But that was only the beginning. Through the 1500s, epidemic after epidemic of European diseases swept north into North America and then to the Atlantic coast. Indians died by the millions; sometimes whole villages were destroyed and once-mighty tribes were broken. When the Puritans arrived to establish their little colony in Plymouth in 1620, they found a place empty of people, ready for European settlements. Although the figures are debated, it is agreed that European dis-

Some Disease Definitions

communicable: spread from person to person only by physical contact

contagious: spread from person to person in any manner, such as by physical contact, body wastes, or droplets in the air from coughing and sneezing

endemic: constantly present in a community or population, but affecting only a small number of people at a time

epidemic: affecting a large number of people in a community, a nation, or a population at once

immune: unable to catch a particular disease

infectious: caused by an invading pathogen, usually a fungus, bacteria, or virus, which attacks an organ or system of the body

inoculate: to give a person a minor case of a disease in order to produce an immunity

pandemic: an epidemic that spreads to a large part of the world

zoonosis: an illness that can pass from an animal to a human

eases, especially smallpox, reduced the Indian population to a fraction of what it had been before Columbus. Without question, smallpox and other European infectious diseases were critical in opening the way for the European conquest of the Americas and the creation of the United States that eventually followed.

Smallpox, then, has played a major role in shaping the history of Earth. It had the power not only to claim the lives of individuals, but to bring down empires, even whole cultures. Even as late as two hundred years ago, it was viewed as a scourge—feared, hated, and always there ready to strike without warning. The idea that it might someday be wiped out seemed to most people impossible.

We must remember that, even as late as the eighteenth century, nobody in the world had much of an idea what caused disease, from the simplest headache to the deadliest of infections. Various people had learned, through trial and error, to cure a few illnesses.

Going back to the Stone Age, there is evidence of head operations, and humans certainly knew how to set broken bones thousands of years ago. Various folk medicines, using herbs, berries, grasses, and tree bark, had long been in use. Some of them worked; most didn't. It was known, for example, that an infusion, or liquid, made from the bark of the cinchona tree was helpful in warding off fevers; and as we have seen, lime juice helped prevent scurvy. But nobody knew why any of these things worked, and in the face of most diseases even the wisest doctors were helpless.

Thus the source of smallpox also remained unknown. Incredible as it may seem, even into the nineteenth century many doctors and scientists did not believe that infectious diseases were contagious. We will learn more about this later. But one thing was clear: if you lived through an attack of smallpox, you would never get it again. That had been understood for a long time. Far back in history people at various times and places had inoculated themselves with the disease, usually by rubbing some of the pus from a smallpox victim into a small scratch in their own skin. With luck, they would get a mild case of smallpox and then be immune from the disease for the rest of their lives.

Nonetheless, the idea of giving yourself such a terrible disease was not a pleasant one, and inoculation had never been widely practiced. It was certainly not accepted in Europe. Then, an eighteenth-century Englishwoman named Mary Wortley Montagu got involved. Lady Mary, as she was generally known, "never thought, spoke, acted or dressed like anybody else." As a girl, she had taught herself Latin and literature at a time when few women were educated. She later became a great friend of major literary figures, including Dr. Samuel Johnson, perhaps the most important literary influence of his day, and the great poet Alexander Pope. Lady Mary was thought to be scandalous by many people, but she commanded public attention.

In 1715 Lady Mary contracted a mild case of smallpox. Luckily her skin was left unmarked, but she lost her eyebrows, which gave her a slightly staring look. By coincidence, two years later her husband was sent to Constantinople (now called Istanbul) as British ambassador to Turkey. In those days when travel was much slower and more difficult, Turkey seemed to the English a strange and distant land. Lady Mary wrote long, amusing letters to her friends back home about the manners and customs of the Turks. Among other things, she noted that inoculation against smallpox was fairly common. She wrote, "People send to one another to know if any of their family has a mind to have the smallpox: they make up parties for this purpose, and when they are met (commonly fifteen or sixteen together), the old woman comes with a nutshell of matter of the best sort of smallpox, and asks what veins you please to have opened. . . ."

Lady Mary had her son inoculated (she of course had had the disease and did not need inoculation). When she returned to London a year later, she began urging English people to adopt the practice of inoculation. As an aristocrat she had contacts at the court—she knew King George I. She decided to have her small daughter inoculated. The king was extremely interested to know if inoculation was safe and had four famous physicians assigned to keep watch over the child and report the results. The inoculation worked, and Lady Mary began pushing hard to see that the practice was widely adopted. A lot of people accepted the idea and supported her, including the Prince of Wales. But many, probably the majority, were opposed. Most doctors were scornful of inoculation, which they thought dangerous, ineffective, or both. The clergy "descanted from their pulpits on the impiety of those seeking to take events out of the hand of Providence," as one of Lady Mary's friends put it.

A lot of the opposition to smallpox inoculation was mindless, but nonetheless the method did have real problems. For one, sometimes people who were inoculated came down with a case of the disease that was serious enough to kill them. For another, inoculation did not always work. For a third—and this was important—a person who had even a mild case of smallpox was highly contagious and might give the disease to somebody else, especially a family member, who might then get a serious case. Finally, at the time, bloodletting and starving were thought to be cures for many illnesses. People who were to be inoculated were sometimes bled, starved, or both in order to prepare them for the disease. This only left them weakened and more vulnerable to coming down with a serious case of it. Inoculation was not without its risks.

One person who happened to be particularly aware of the dangers of inoculation was a boy growing up in Berkeley, Gloucester, England, not far from the River Severn, which separates England from Wales. It was a rural area filled with cattle, sheep, horses, woods, and fields of grain. The boy was Edward Jenner. His father was the local minister at a time when ministers were the leading figures in towns and villages and often set the tone for the populace. Edward's father kept up with the times and had Edward inoculated against smallpox. The boy underwent a course of bleeding and starvation. The ordeal was very painful for him and left him feeling unwell for months. He grew up no friend of inoculation.

Edward Jenner was a born naturalist, a child who liked exploring the fields, streams, and woods around his home to study the flowers and the animals. Throughout his life Jenner continued to have a strong interest in nature: he turned down an opportunity to work in London with a famous physician in order to live in his native countryside. There he made a long series of nature studies, including trying to learn how animals could hibernate for months without eating, a great mystery at the time.

Jenner's interest in nature led him into biology and then medicine. He studied in London, then in the 1770s returned to his beloved Berkeley to build his practice. It was, as we have seen, farm country. There was among the local people a belief, which existed elsewhere in England too, that anyone who had had a mild, rather common disease called cowpox never seemed to catch smallpox.

Cowpox was a disease that left sores on the udders of cows. Diseased or not, cows had to be milked twice a day; otherwise the milk built up, which was not only painful for the cow, it could cause it to have health problems as well. So the people milking infected cows often got cowpox, which caused pustules to appear on their hands. The disease usually ran its course in a short time.

By the time Jenner set up his practice in Berkeley, it had been more than fifty years since Lady Mary Wortley Montagu had begun promoting inoculation. It was no longer a novelty. But Jenner was still not a fan. Then, in 1778, there was a smallpox epidemic in his area, and people came to him demanding to be inoculated. Jenner had to comply. In the course of tending to his patients, he noticed that in a few people the inoculation did not take. He knew this because usually the inoculated person ran a fever and had pustules surrounding the point of the inoculation. But these few people showed no such signs. He questioned them and discovered that they were, like many people in the area, dairy workers who regularly milked cows.

Jenner knew of the folk belief that cowpox prevented smallpox. His curiosity was aroused, so he inoculated these people again. There was still no reaction. This was not normal, and Jenner began to believe that perhaps the folktale was true. If so, was it possible that the terrible scourge of smallpox could be brought to an end?

Jenner was a good scientist, and he went about his work carefully. First he made a study of cowpox, questioning milkers, examining infected cows, and treating people who had the disease. Very soon he realized that while most people who had contracted cowpox did not get smallpox later, some did. Cowpox did not seem to be an effective preventative in every case. Why?

For several years he struggled with the question, studying it from all

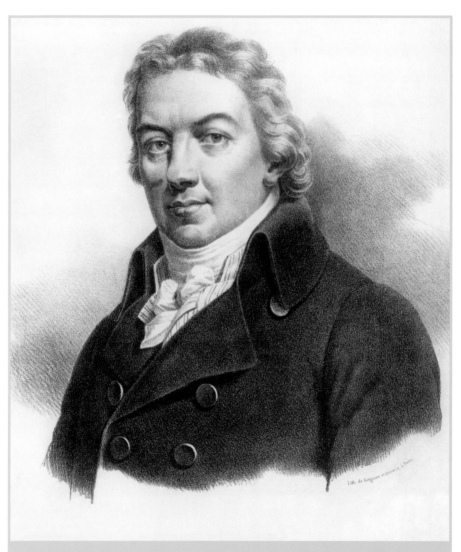

EDWARD JENNER WAS NOT THE FIRST TO REALIZE THE LINK BETWEEN COWPOX AND SMALLPOX. RURAL ENGLISH DAIRY WORKERS LEARNED THAT HAVING COWPOX OFTEN CREATED A FUTURE IMMUNITY TO SMALLPOX. BUT JENNER WAS THE FIRST TO PROVE THE CONNECTION BETWEEN THE TWO. HIS WORK PAVED THE WAY FOR DISCOVERING SIMILAR DEFENSES AGAINST OTHER INFECTIOUS DISEASES.

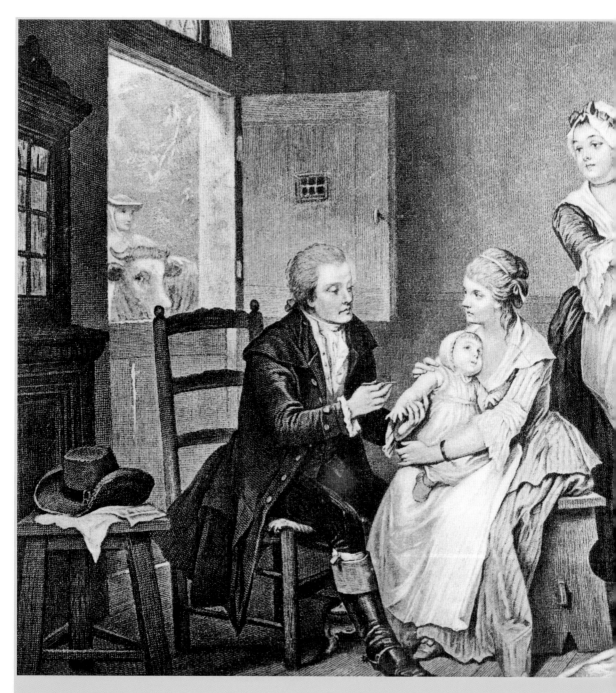

EDWARD JENNER TURNED TO LOCAL DAIRY WORKERS TO TEST AND SUPPORT HIS THEORIES OF INOCULATION. HERE AN INFANT IS VACCINATED WITH COWPOX TAKEN FROM ITS MOTHER, WHO CONTRACTED THE DISEASE WHILE MILKING. THE POSSIBLE CULPRIT, A COW FROM A NEARBY FARM, PEERS INTO THE SITTING ROOM IN THIS COPPER ENGRAVING FROM THE 1800S.

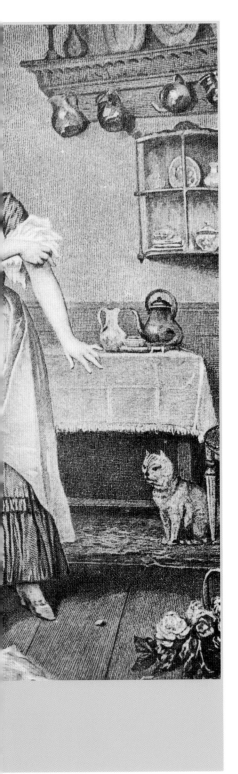

sides. Then, in 1780, he came across one of those cases—a man sick with smallpox, who insisted that he had previously had cowpox. Jenner questioned the man closely: when had he had cowpox and how had he contracted it? Suddenly a thought occurred to him. There was a disease common among farmworkers that resembled cowpox in certain ways. It was an affliction of the heels of horses, known among farmers as grease. Sometimes farmhands caught it too.

Now, Jenner asked, had this particular farmhand noticed cases of grease among the horses he had worked with? He had indeed. So perhaps he had not had cowpox after all, but grease. This would explain the cases of people who got smallpox despite having had cowpox: they had never had cowpox in the first place, but grease instead.

It was an important insight, and it was a lesson for the future: again and again in the fight against infectious diseases, researchers have thought they were dealing with one disease, when in fact there was more than one present. For example, as we will eventually see, a serious mistake would be made in the effort to discover the polio vaccine before it was realized that there were several strains of the disease.

Jenner then went about determining the difference between grease and cowpox, and by 1782 he was able to differentiate between "true" versus "spurious" cowpox. He thought that he would then be able to proceed toward a *vaccine*, a word that did not yet exist. But in 1791, when he was still testing his theory, he discovered that some of those who had "true" cowpox still came down with smallpox. The number was not large, but it was enough to suggest that cowpox might not be the preventative he had hoped.

Once again he struggled, this time for two years. Then, in the course of examining an animal with cowpox, he had a crucial insight: the strength, or potency, of the cowpox might be a factor. Once more he patiently began his studies. He now discovered that cowpox immunized people against smallpox only when the cowpox was at peak strength in the cow. At other times it was not potent enough to create an immunity.

Of course neither Jenner nor anyone else knew anything about the body's immune system. All Jenner had was his one predictable result: you didn't get smallpox if you had had "true" cowpox at the right potency beforehand. But Jenner's theory was based on interviews, not trials. He had built it from the medical histories people had given him. That was not going to convince the medical world; nor, Jenner realized, should he let it convince him either. He would have to make a trial.

But there were several problems. For one, at a time before refrigeration it was not possible to store smallpox or cowpox "matter" for future experiments. Jenner could only make a trial during an outbreak of cowpox.

A second problem was ethical: could he in good conscience deliberately infect someone with cowpox, to say nothing of smallpox? Today such an experiment would not be permitted. Jenner undoubtedly felt that risking the life of a few people on the chance of eliminating smallpox was worth it. Besides, he was convinced that he was right—the experiment would be safe.

In May 1796 there was another outbreak of cowpox, and Jenner had

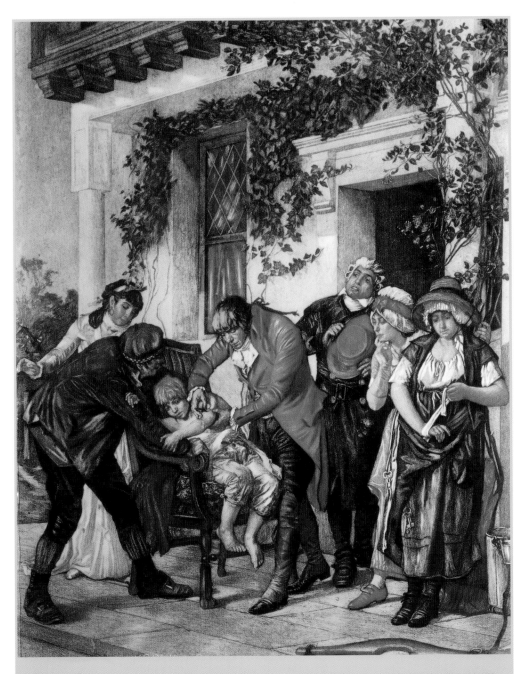

EDWARD JENNER TESTED HIS THEORIES OF SMALLPOX ON AN EIGHT-YEAR-OLD GUINEA PIG NAMED JAMES PHIPPS. THIS BRAVE BOY BECAME A MEDICAL HERO FOR HIS ROLE IN THE DISCOVERY OF SMALLPOX INOCULATION.

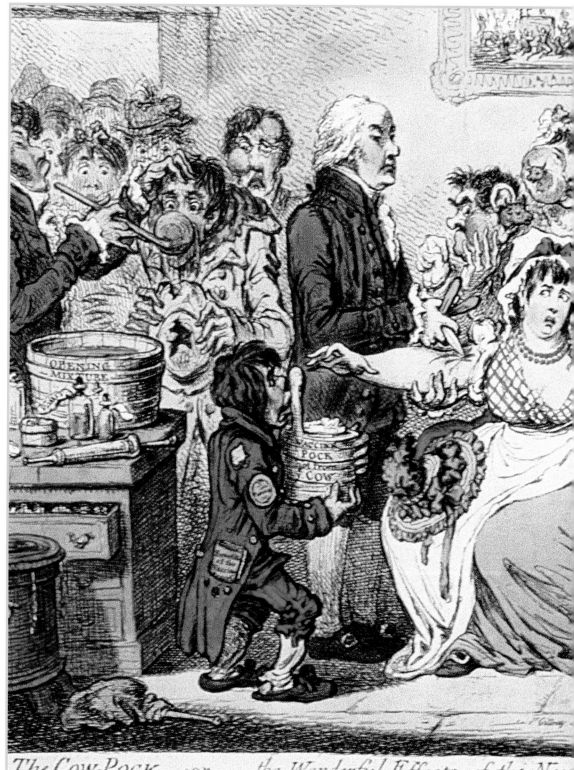

The Cow-Pock __ or __ the Wonderful Effects of the New

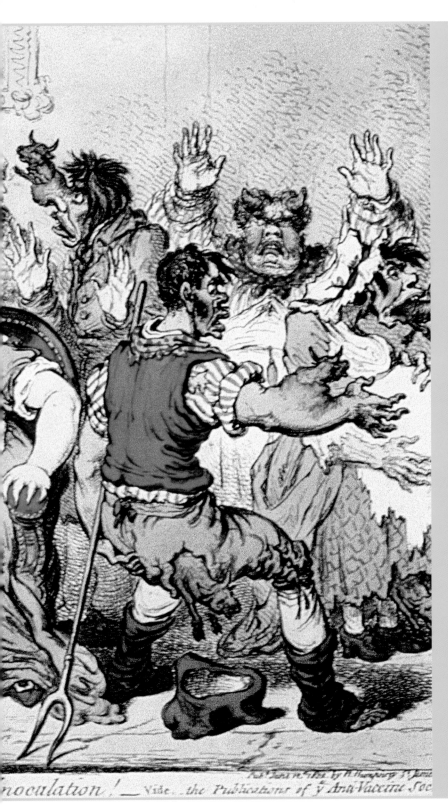

inoculation! _ Vide the Publications of ỹ Anti-Vaccine Soc

For some time, Edward Jenner's theory only met with criticism. The English satirical artist James Gilray created in this cartoon a vision of the possible effects of cow-pox inoculation.

41

his opportunity. For the experiment, he now needed a subject who had never had either smallpox or cowpox, and that would most likely be a child. He turned to a laborer named Phipps who had done some work for him over the years and who had an eight-year-old son named James who had never had either disease. He discussed the matter with the boy's father. His wife raised vigorous objections, but Phipps trusted Jenner and gave his assent. So Jenner brought to Phipps's cottage a dairy woman named Sarah Nelmes, who was suffering from cowpox. He made a 2.5-inch (6.4-cm) incision in the arm of young James Phipps and smeared in the cut some pus from the infected woman. James became ill with cowpox briefly and then recovered. So far, so good.

Now came the critical and dangerous part of the experiment. From a smallpox sufferer in the area, he took some pus and inoculated James Phipps with it. For two weeks he watched and waited. By the end of a month, James showed no signs of smallpox, not even the pustules that typically appeared around the point of inoculation. It was, after almost twenty years, a magnificent achievement.

With his proof in hand, Jenner wrote a paper and submitted it to Sir Joseph Banks, head of the Royal Society, at the time the leading scientific society in England and probably the world. Banks refused the paper: Jenner's evidence was not strong enough, he felt, especially to support a theory that ran counter to the accepted wisdom. So in 1798, now certain that he was right, Jenner repeated the experiments on several more subjects, including his eleven-month-old son, Robert. (Because Jenner had been inoculated, he could not use himself as a subject.) The trial was again a success. He wrote a new paper and, bypassing the Royal Society, published it himself. For the paper he coined the word *vaccine*, from the Latin word for cow, *vacca*. He sent copies of the paper to well-known scientists and doctors in the United States and Europe.

Inevitably, as had been the case with inoculation, there was opposition: it seemed unnatural to many people to infect somebody with the disease of an animal. Again many religious people believed that vaccination was contrary to the wishes of God. But slowly people accepted the idea. It was particularly well received in the United States where smallpox continued to be a deadly disease among the Indians, many of whom lived in close contact with whites. Americans were well aware of its dangers, and interest in the new vaccine grew. In time, vaccination against smallpox became commonplace in the Western world. But it would be a long time before Jenner's dream of eradicating the disease would be realized.

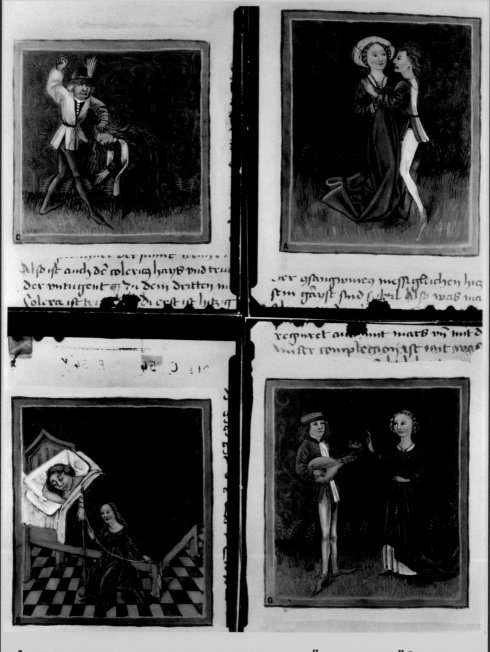

IN MEDIEVAL TIMES, MANY PEOPLE BELIEVED THEY POSSESSED "TEMPERAMENTS." IF AN EXCESS OF TEMPERAMENT GATHERED IN AN INDIVIDUAL, PROBLEMS WOULD RESULT. THIS ILLUSTRATION SHOWS THE FOUR TEMPERAMENTS: CHOLERIC, MELANCHOLIC, PHLEGMATIC, AND SANGUINE. WE STILL USE THESE WORDS TO DENOTE ANGER, SADNESS, CALM, AND OPTIMISM.

＊ T H R E E ＊

Death Invisible

In the 1600s a Dutch cloth merchant named Antonie van Leeuwenhoek, for his own amusement, began to grind lenses for eyeglasses and the simple microscopes of the time. Leeuwenhoek became a master of what was then a difficult art. With his high-quality lenses he started exploring the invisible world around him, examining the innards of animals, rainwater, and other subjects. He soon found a vast world of tiny creatures inhabiting the bits and pieces of things that he put under his microscope. He called them animalcules. Some were shaped like rods, some like fishhooks, others like coiled springs.

Many of them seemed to be able to swim or move around. In the 1670s Leeuwenhoek sent drawings of these tiny creatures to the British Royal Society. There was a lot of interest in Leeuwenhoek's animalcules, both among scientists and amateur naturalists. But nobody knew what to make of them, and they remained in the minds of most people a curious, yet not terribly significant part of nature.

Nonetheless, there was an awareness that small creatures seemed almost invariably to appear on rotting fruit, vegetables, and meat—dead organic matter. There were not only Leeuwenhoek's animalcules, but also much larger creatures easily visible to the naked eye, such as flies and maggots. Why did such creatures appear so frequently on decaying matter, and where did they come from? There was no explanation, and it was generally conceded that they appeared spontaneously on their own, somehow forming from the putrefying material around them. This theory of spontaneous generation was generally accepted. And, since the spontaneously generated creatures usually appeared on dead and decaying matter, they seemed somehow to be linked to illness and death.

But the theory did not explain the origin of infectious diseases such as smallpox, cholera, and the plague, which also seemed to appear out of midair. How was it that the people in one house, one street, or one town might suffer heavy losses from a certain disease, while those in a neighboring place went unscathed? It seemed clear to a lot of people that such diseases were "catching"—they could be passed from one person to another. Nobody knew quite how this worked, but the general idea seemed obvious. For that reason some towns and cities imposed quarantines of various types to prevent the spread of contagious diseases. Some places might, for example, prevent ships carrying sick passengers or crew members from landing, forcing them to anchor in the harbor until the ill were either cured or dead and their bodies disposed of. Or they might require sick people to stay in their houses until they recovered or died.

But not everybody believed that infectious diseases were catching. A better explanation, they thought, was that such illnesses were caused by something in the air, an invisible presence often termed a miasma. It seemed that the miasma drifted with the air from street to street, from town to town, missing some while infecting others. What, precisely, this miasma consisted of, nobody was sure, but it probably was like some kind of poison.

The miasma theory of disease was widely accepted, especially among doctors, scientists, and scholars. It seemed to them to make the most sense; but there was a second more practical reason for believing it. Quarantines were a nuisance, hard to enforce, and costly for some

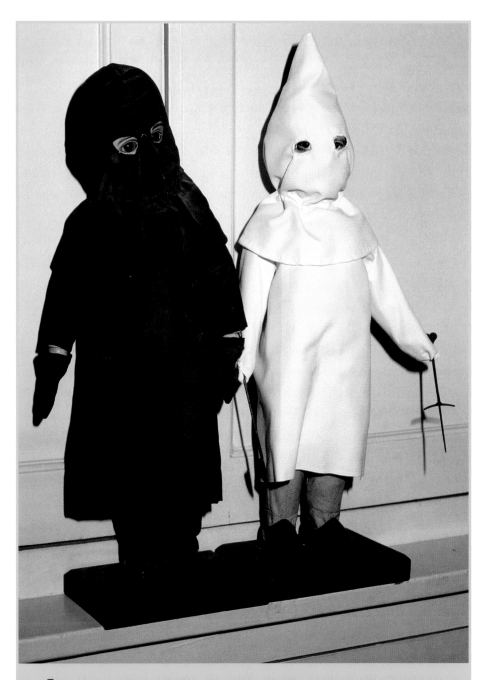

EVEN AFTER IT WAS RECOGNIZED THAT DISEASE COULD BE SPREAD FROM PERSON TO PERSON OR VIA A MIASMA, IT WAS STILL NOT KNOWN HOW. THESE COSTUMES, DISPLAYED IN THE PASTEUR INSTITUTE IN PARIS, FRANCE, ARE MINIATURE VERSIONS OF THE ONES WORN IN THE FOURTEENTH CENTURY TO WARD OFF PLAGUE.

people. A ship held up in a harbor and unable to unload its cargo cost the ship's owners money and was a problem for the traders and merchants who had counted on receiving the goods. If disease was not passed from person to person, but was spread by a miasma, there was little point in imposing quarantines. There were, then, good financial reasons for believing in the miasma theory of disease. Edward Jenner may have shown that vaccination would immunize a person from smallpox, but he had not shown how smallpox was spread. There was nothing in Jenner's work to negate the miasma theory of disease.

Then, in 1822, a boy named Louis Pasteur was born in eastern France. He grew up in the Jura Mountains, not far from the Swiss border. His father, a tanner, had fought in the imperial armies of Napoleon and imbued young Louis with a fiery patriotism that would last throughout his life. The boy was determined, proud, and obviously very intelligent. He studied art in school but, although he showed promise, he eventually switched to chemistry. His brilliance in his studies attracted the attention of important scientists, and in his midtwenties he did some extremely important work in the study of crystals.

In 1854 Pasteur was appointed head of a science department at a university in Lille in western France. Lille was an industrial area, and it was understood that university scientists would help local industry in whatever ways they could. One of the main industries around Lille was wine making and more generally the manufacture of alcohol. Pasteur started a university course in alcohol making and in his spare time consulted with wine and alcohol manufacturers about their problems.

The making of wine, beer, and the alcohol derived from such products involved fermentation, a process that had been of intense interest for at least 2,000 years. It was known that fermentation was necessary to turn grape juice into wine and to make bread rise. It also was involved in the souring of milk and was somehow related to the putrefaction of organic material—the very material on which flies and maggots seemed to generate spontaneously. To us fermentation might seem a dull topic. To Pasteur and the people of his time, it was a mystery, basic to some very primary biological processes.

Pasteur set out to decipher fermentation. He was motivated, like any good scientist, in part by intellectual curiosity. But he also knew that if he came to understand the process better, he might help the local wine makers avoid losing those batches of wine that somehow turned sour or cloudy and thus could not be sold.

As is often the case with important scientific breakthroughs, Pasteur's work on fermentation followed a tortuous path, complete with disappointments, false leads, and new beginnings. But in the course of his studies, he began to notice in his microscopic examination of fermenting material tiny creatures that moved and reproduced by dividing. His mind made an important leap: these little creatures were responsible for fermentation. And he drew a second conclusion: these creatures were not generated spontaneously in the fermenting substance but had somehow fallen into it from the air. They were, of course, Leeuwenhoek's animalcules.

He began experimenting to prove this theory. In one experiment he drew juice from a grape with a hypodermic needle in such a way that it never touched the skin of the grape. This juice would not ferment. In another experiment he covered the budding grapes with cloth so they were not touched by air. Juice from these grapes would not ferment either.

From these and other experiments, Pasteur learned that yeast was necessary to most types of fermentation. He then showed that when certain of Leeuwenhoek's animalcules were present during the fermentation process, the wine, beer, or whatever was being manufactured might be spoiled. He also discovered that if the material being fermented, such as grape juice, was heated to a certain point, the little creatures would be killed and there would be no spoilage. This process, still used today in the preparation of various foods, is called pasteurization.

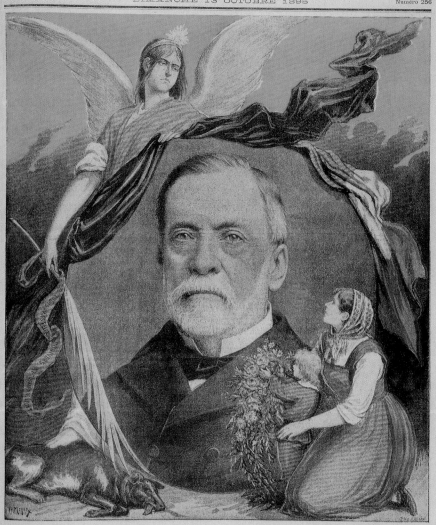

A LOUIS PASTEUR

As a scientist, Louis Pasteur understood that experiments needed to be performed with care, with nothing left to chance. His discoveries won him a measure of public acclaim. At the time of his death, a leading French magazine made him its cover story.

Pasteur now tackled the theory of spontaneous generation with a demonstration that is still used in biology classes. He put fermentable juice in glass flasks and sealed them. As long as they were sealed off from the air, the juice would not ferment. However when he exposed the juice to air, fermentation began. Air, or something in the air, was necessary to the process. Which was it? Next he repeated the experiment, but this time he heated the necks of some of the flasks and bent them into the shape of a swan's neck. When he unsealed the flasks, the juice still did not ferment, even though it was exposed to the air. Pasteur reasoned that it did not ferment because the tiny creatures in the air ran into the walls of the curved spout and stuck there before they could reach the juice. This, for Pasteur, was his evidence: air alone did not cause fermentation. It was caused instead by his little creatures, which were not generated spontaneously in the fermenting liquid but were suspended in the air. Pasteur's creatures were, of course, bacteria.

Pasteur then made another imaginative leap from fermentation to putrefaction. Once again studying his subjects under the microscope, he deduced that microorganisms—tiny living creatures—were responsible for breaking down dead matter into its basic elements through its decay and eventual dissolution. This was an essential biological process, for only when dead matter was broken down could the building blocks out of which new life was made be recycled.

Pasteur was then asked to look into a disease that at the time was afflicting France's vital silk-making industry. This was the kind of practical work that Pasteur liked because if he could find the answers, they would be of immediate benefit to people and not so incidentally to his beloved France. He knew that he then had to look for some kind of microorganism, and after a good deal of searching, he found two microscopic parasites that were responsible for the silkworm disease. He then showed silkworm farmers procedures that would keep the microbe, or disease-causing microorganism, from infecting the worms,

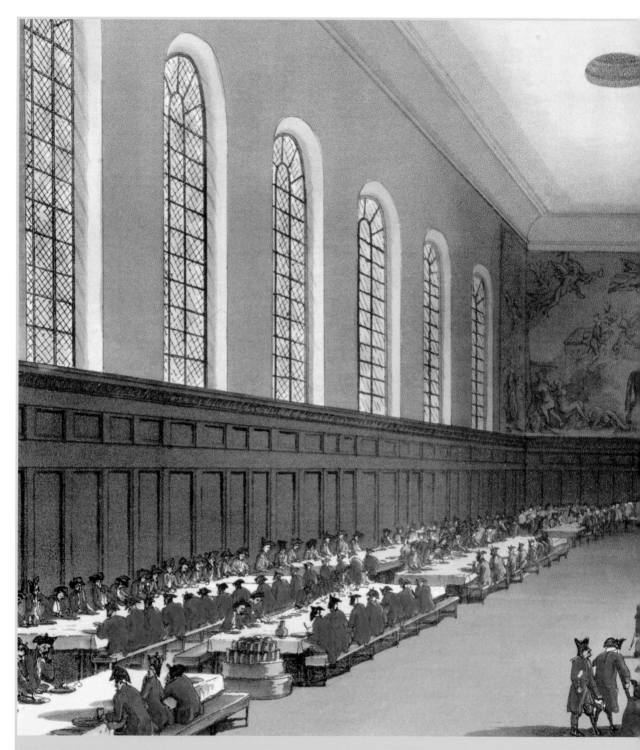

EVEN AS LATE AS 1810 IT WAS NOT KNOWN THAT UNSANITARY CONDITIONS HELPED SPREAD DISEASE. CHELSEA HOSPITAL IN LONDON, ENGLAND, WAS STAFFED BY DOCTORS WHO WORE ORDINARY STREET CLOTHES. PATIENTS WERE NOT ISOLATED FROM EACH OTHER BUT GROUPED CLOSE ENOUGH TO SPREAD DISEASE AMONG THEM.

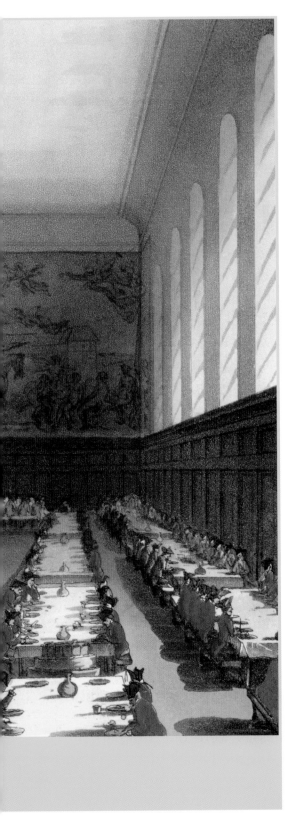

and very shortly the industry rebounded.

The important point was that Pasteur was now demonstrating a key principle of modern medicine, the germ theory of infectious disease. The term *germ* had been around for a while, vaguely defined as some kind of small body that could eventually grow into something else, as a seed becomes a flower. The term then came to mean any of a variety of small pathogens (what later became known as bacteria or viruses) that cause infectious diseases. Disease, Pasteur concluded, was not spread by that vaguely defined miasma so many believed in, but was carried by germs. There seemed to be a huge number of them, and he was able to show experimentally that some needed air in order to survive, while others could survive only without air. The germ theory of disease states that a given disease is caused by a given pathogen: find that particular pathogen and somehow neutralize it, and the disease will be stopped.

All of this is known to us today, but at the time many people, including leading scientists and medical people, had trouble accepting it. As ever, entrenched ideas were difficult to dis-

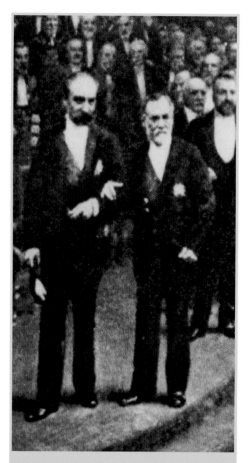

THIS RARE PHOTOGRAPH SHOWS JOSEPH LISTER (LEFT) AND LOUIS PASTEUR TOGETHER. IT WAS TAKEN AT AN EVENT HONORING THESE MEN WHO HAD CONTRIBUTED SO MUCH TO ENDING DEATH CAUSED BY INFECTIOUS DISEASE. LISTER HAD JUST RETIRED FROM TEACHING, AND PASTEUR HAD JUST TURNED SEVENTY.

lodge. People are often reluctant to give up notions and principles they have always held to be true, and many in the scientific establishment fought against Pasteur's new theories.

Yet most doctors had long been appalled by the aftereffects of operations. Time after time an operation was successful, but the patient died of some infection. With no understanding of bacteria or even that any such thing existed, hospitals, including operating rooms, were run without any thought to cleanliness. A doctor might operate on a patient, then perform an autopsy on someone who had just died, then head for another operation, without changing his clothes or even washing his hands. The effects were, inevitably, tragic.

The first glimmer of sense came to a young doctor named Ignaz Semmelweis, a Hungarian who had moved to Vienna as a student. He observed that at one of two obstetric clinics in Vienna many of the women died of complications of childbirth, whereas in the other one many survived. What was the difference? Semmelweis noticed that in the less deadly clinic only midwives aided in childbirth, whereas in the other, more deadly one, medical students helped. "Since death came with the medical students, they should be banished from the delivery room," he argued. The death rate of the second clinic immediately fell.

Semmelweis concluded that the illnesses were due to "particles" that were present in the operating room or were brought in by the doctors themselves. He then began insisting that doctors scrub their hands with a chlorine solution. The mortality rate at clinics that followed this practice dropped to less than 2 percent overnight.

That should have been enough for most people, but it wasn't. Opposition to Semmelweis's ideas was powerful. Older, more experienced doctors were determined to stick by the methods and ideas that had become ingrained in them and refused to use the scrubbing procedure. It is also true that Semmelweis was not by nature tactful and sometimes alienated people who might otherwise have come over to his side. In any case the rejection of his ideas crushed him. He left Vienna, and his work was forgotten until many years later, when he began to receive credit for his pioneering efforts.

It was left to the Englishman Joseph Lister to win the battle against operating-room infection. Troubled as he was by the death rate after operations, he was on the lookout for a cause. He began to notice that people who had broken a bone that had not penetrated the skin usually healed without problems. In cases where the accident had caused a flesh wound as well as a broken bone, there were likely to be complications. Something, clearly, was getting into the wound. At this point he came across Pasteur's work on putrefaction. That seemed similar to infection, and Lister immediately concluded that bacteria were responsible for the infections he was seeing in his patients. He eventually settled on a solution of carbolic acid as a sterilizing agent and soon began reducing the rate of operating deaths in his hospital. As usual, a lot of people opposed his new method; but statistics piled up showing that Lister's system of sterilization dramatically reduced hospital deaths, and gradually sanitation became routine in hospitals—and, indeed, in all medical practice.

By the 1870s the germ theory of disease was gradually establishing itself. Pasteur was seen as the leading scientist in France—indeed, in all of Europe. He had a flair for publicity and usually managed to draw attention to his work. Nonetheless he was a brilliant scientist, always exceedingly careful to check everything thoroughly, and gifted with one insight after the next that usually led him in the right direction.

After Pasteur's success in aiding both the wine-making and silk-worm industries, the French minister of agriculture asked him for help in preventing two other serious agricultural diseases: anthrax and chicken cholera. Pasteur was confident that he could find vaccines for both diseases. His first breakthrough came with chicken cholera. According to one story, in the summer of 1879, in the midst of work on chicken cholera, Pasteur's lab closed down for the traditional long French summer vacation. When the lab reopened, Pasteur and his assistants noticed that some chicken cholera bacteria that had been left in the lab could no longer infect experimental animals with the disease. It had somehow become weaker. Why? They could not answer that question. The researchers tried to strengthen the bacteria. Then they injected it into several chickens. This batch of bacteria still would not kill. So they gave up on the older batch and injected the same chickens with a dose of fresh bacteria. They were startled to discover that the ones that had been given the old batch survived the second, fresh batch, while those that had not been inoculated with the old batch died.

Pasteur's imagination immediately turned to Jenner and cowpox: there was something about the old, weaker batch of bacteria that made the chickens immune. He and his assistants began searching for ways to weaken chicken cholera bacteria. Eventually they concluded that exposure to the oxygen in the air for a period of time weakened the bacteria.

Pasteur now began injecting chickens with this attenuated bacteria and discovered that it did indeed make them immune. The word *immunity* dates back to an older English one that meant exempt; you might be immune from paying a certain tax. Now it was applied to medicine and the new science of immunology, which Louis Pasteur was doing a lot to create.

Chicken cholera was a disease that affected chicken farmers, but did not figure largely in the public imagination. Anthrax did: not only did it kill a lot of animals, but it could also cause humans to die quickly and unpleasantly. Pasteur now began looking for an anthrax vaccine.

Others had been working along the same lines. Among them was a German, Robert Koch, who would prove almost as important as Pasteur in the search for vaccines. Several years earlier Koch had identified the anthrax bacterium and learned how to culture it. With this as a starting point, Pasteur set about finding ways to attenuate it. He was in the midst of his experiments when another scientist named Toussaint announced that he had the secret: you could attenuate the anthrax bacterium by heating it to a certain point.

Pasteur was astonished that this young scientist had beaten him to it, and remained somewhat unbelieving. He and his assistants repeated Toussaint's experiments and discovered that heating attenuated the bacterium only temporarily; given time, it returned to full strength. However, Pasteur discovered that if he heated the bacterium to a specific

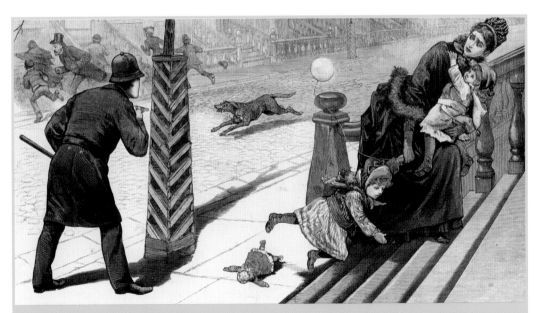

THE THREAT OF THE SPREAD OF RABIES HAS ALWAYS SPARKED FEAR. IN THIS NINETEENTH-CENTURY ENGRAVING, PEOPLE IN NEW YORK CITY ARE SHOWN FLEEING FROM A DOG DURING WHAT WAS THOUGHT TO BE A MAD DOG "EPIDEMIC."

temperature and then exposed it to oxygen, he could attenuate it permanently. He now had his anthrax vaccine.

The news rapidly spread. Officials, farmers, and journalists started demanding a field test. A veterinarian and writer named Rossignal who had a farm near the town of Melun, not far outside Paris, offered his farm for the field tests. Local farmers volunteered to contribute sheep and cattle for the experiment.

Pasteur felt that he was being rushed into the trial before he was fully ready. He wanted to do further testing of his methods first. But, pushed and prodded, he finally agreed. Fortunately at the last minute two of his assistants worked out a better system for attenuating the vaccine with carbolic acid and convinced Pasteur to use this approach instead.

Still, Pasteur was worried. But he had to go ahead. On May 5, 1881, Pasteur and his assistants arrived at the farm near Melun to begin the first injections. He found a huge crowd there. It was like a country fair, said one historian.

There were sixty experimental animals, both sheep and cattle. Twenty-five of them were to be vaccinated, twenty-five left unvaccinated, and ten left out of the experiment altogether to act as controls. The vaccinated animals would be given two shots about two weeks apart; and then after two weeks both the vaccinated and unvaccinated animals would be given the deadly anthrax bacteria. There was great speculation in the press. At this point believers in the vaccine were in the minority; most people could not conceive of how such a thing would work. Inwardly Pasteur had his worries, but he maintained a calm exterior.

Three and a half weeks later, on May 31, the anthrax was injected into the fifty animals. The ten controls were not infected with anything; if they sickened and died, it would show that the experimental animals might have already had the disease.

Now there was nothing to do but wait. Within a day the sheep that had not been vaccinated began to sicken, and within two days they were dying. But it also appeared that some of the vaccinated sheep were growing sick too. Pasteur returned to Paris and waited. Even his faith began to waver. Then, on the morning of June 2, a telegram from Melun arrived: the unvaccinated animals were all dead or dying; the vaccinated ones were alive and healthy. The field trial was a "tremendous success." Pasteur had proven that his anthrax vaccine worked. Over the next ten years, 3.5 million sheep and a half million cattle were vaccinated and only 1 percent of them died.

Pasteur next turned his attention to rabies. In fact rabies, while exceedingly deadly, had never caused a great many deaths, perhaps a few hundred a year in France, as opposed to thousands, even tens of thousands of deaths from diseases such as cholera and smallpox. But rabies had a grip on the human imagination: the image of the mad, slavering wolf or dog racing through the village streets snarling and slashing at people had been a staple of folklore for millennia. Furthermore death from rabies was not only intensely painful, but was protracted, lasting in some cases several weeks. Particularly sinister was one symptom of the disease, hydrophobia, or fear of water. Dogs or humans afflicted with rabies would be ravenously thirsty, but would recoil from water, which was too painful to swallow.

At the outset Pasteur took it for granted that rabies was caused by a microbe of some kind, but previous researchers had not been able to find a rabies bacterium, and neither could Pasteur. The process of getting pure strains of bacteria for experiments or making vaccines requires filtering them out of the liquid they're found in. By Pasteur's time, filters fine enough to capture something as small as bacteria had been developed. But whatever was causing rabies was so small that it passed through the filters of the day. It would eventually turn out that these creatures were so small that they could live inside bacteria. Although they could not be seen, Pasteur knew that they had to exist; he called them *viruses*, a term that had been in use for a while to denote a mysterious disease-causing agent.

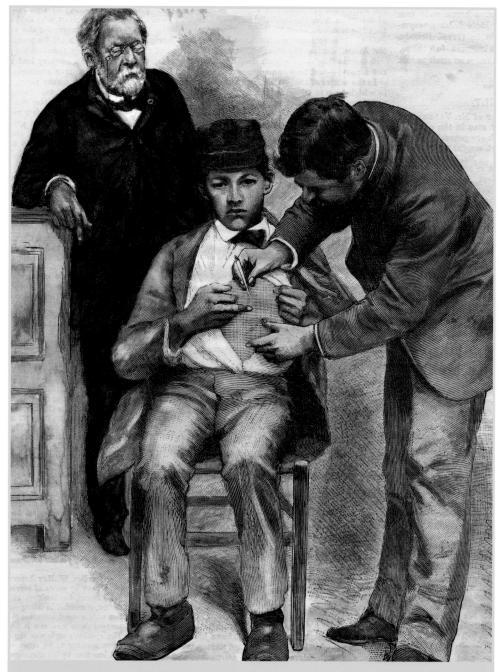

THIS PAINTING SHOWS LOUIS PASTEUR LOOKING ON, AS A MAN IS INOCULATED AGAINST RABIES.

Pasteur decided that he would not try to identify and isolate the virus that caused rabies; that would have to come some other time. He would instead move directly toward making some kind of vaccine, presumably by attenuating the virus. For several years he experimented on a variety of animals, especially dogs and rabbits, trying to find a way to attenuate the rabies virus, but the secret eluded him. Then one day he noticed that one of the associates in his lab, Emil Roux, was performing an experiment that involved drying the marrow of the spinal cord of a rabbit that had been infected with rabies. Pasteur had always been careful to credit his assistants for their help in his work, but a certain competitiveness had developed between Pasteur and Roux. Pasteur adopted Roux's idea of drying spine marrow to produce an attenuated rabies virus without asking Roux about it. Roux, bitter and angry, dropped his work on rabies.

Pasteur then had another idea. Unlike smallpox and the plague, which killed within a few days, rabies took a long time to develop in the human body—sometimes weeks. Furthermore the victim almost always knew when rabies had been contracted, because it began with a dramatic event, like a dog bite. If the disease took so long to develop, might it not be possible to create a vaccine that would attack rabies and overpower it in its early stages, while it was still weak?

It must be understood that at this stage nobody, not even Pasteur, understood how immunity worked. Pasteur was making educated guesses about a complex subject. But the idea was certainly worth trying because if it worked, it would end a great deal of suffering and death.

The experiments Pasteur and his assistants began were exceedingly dangerous, for it meant working with rabid dogs often howling with rage in their cages. In some of this work the experimenters brought a pistol into the lab with them. If something went wrong —if one of the researchers was bitten by a rabid dog, or cut himself with a scalpel, the other was supposed to shoot the victim in the head. But despite the difficulties, the experiments proceeded, and by 1885 Pasteur had a vaccine that worked—on dogs.

Trying the vaccine on human beings, however, was another matter. Pasteur was worried, but he knew that eventually the trial would have to be made. There was, in fact, little to lose: people bitten by rabid dogs usually died anyway. People began bringing cases to Pasteur, but always too late; the disease had gone too far for the vaccine to halt it.

Then, in July 1885, Pasteur saw nine-year-old Joseph Meister, the son of a baker, who had been bitten fourteen times by a rabid dog. The dog would have killed him had not a stonemason bearing an iron rod come up and driven the dog off. The boy's wounds were fresh, and Pasteur thought there might be a chance to save him. Over the next ten days, Pasteur gave Joseph the series of shots that he had worked out, each one stronger than the previous one. The boy continued to do well. Pasteur's hopes rose with each succeeding day, and finally he let the boy go home. On the day when it was clear that the boy had been cured, he wrote to Pasteur:

> *Dear Monsieur Pasteur,*
>
> *I am feeling good and I sleep well and I also have good appetite. I had fun in the countryside. I didn't like to go back to Paris.*

Pasteur had conquered rabies.

Pasteur's work with rabies was really the last of his major successes. He was now world famous. Joseph Meister remains a name familiar to any student of medicine. Pasteur kept in touch with the boy and later on got him a job as a guard at the Paris Institute in France. There is, however, a sad ending to Meister's story. Many years later in 1940, when the Germans were occupying Paris during World War II, some German officers wanted to visit Pasteur's grave at the institute. Meister was a patriotic Frenchman. He refused to let the Germans visit Pasteur's grave. But his heart was broken by the presence of the enemy at the institute, and he went home and killed himself.

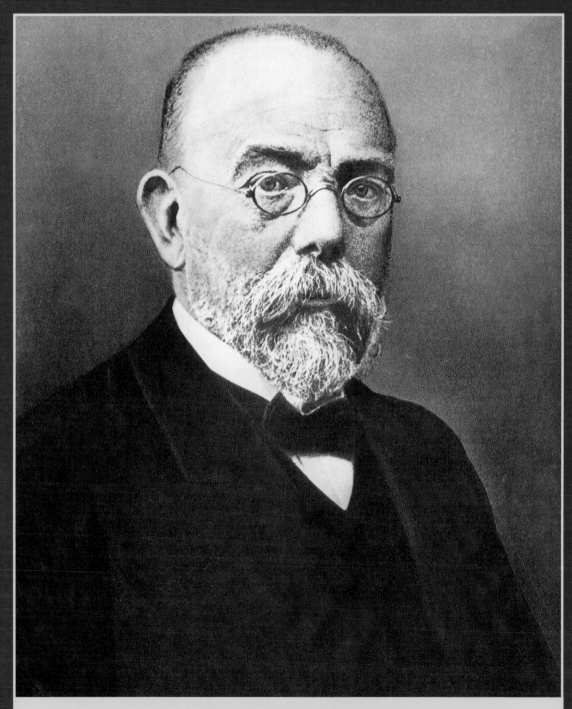

ROBERT KOCH WAS A DETERMINED, DEDICATED SCIENTIST. LIKE LOUIS PASTEUR, HE REPEATED HIS EXPERIMENTS OVER AND OVER TO MAKE SURE HIS RESULTS WERE CORRECT.

Cleaning up the Cities

Louis Pasteur did not develop the anthrax vaccine all by himself. Others contributed, including Koch, Toussaint, and Pasteur's own
assistants. Of these, the most important was the German, Robert Koch.
We must understand that at this time France and Germany were bitter
rivals; Pasteur and Koch were both patriots of their own nations, and
this patriotism strengthened the rivalry between them.

Robert Koch was precisely the opposite kind of person from Louis
Pasteur: where Pasteur was aggressive in promoting his ideas, Koch
held back, endlessly repeating his experiments yet one more time to be
sure. Where Pasteur was eager for rewards and honors, Koch wanted
only to get on with his work. Where Pasteur had been a brilliant student
and had attracted the attention of his superiors from the start, Koch
started his career as a small-town doctor delivering babies and treating
sprained ankles. But Koch, even as he made his daily rounds, was
driven by a desire to do something more interesting and significant. His
chance came when his wife, to assuage his boredom with his small-
town practice, gave him a good quality microscope for his birthday.
Koch taught himself how to use it and then decided to study anthrax
several years before Pasteur turned his attention to the subject.

Koch's work was particularly important in learning ways to manage and control bacteria. Pasteur had generally cultured, or grown, his bacteria in broths of various kinds and then filtered them. The process was always arduous and painstaking.

Koch achieved a breakthrough during the course of his studies of anthrax. One day he noticed that half of a potato somebody had left lying on his lab table showed little spots of different colors on the damp, sliced side. Koch had an insight: the spots might have been caused by bacteria from the air. When he examined them under the microscope, he saw that the spots were indeed bacteria and that each of the differently colored spots had been made by a pure colony of bacteria.

Koch now drew two conclusions. He realized that bacteria cultured in broth could easily mingle with other bacteria, or indeed other material. Bacteria cultured on a solid medium, such as a potato, were less likely to move around. Koch tried culturing bacteria on various jellylike substances. Bacteria, however, could break down gelatin. The wife of one of Koch's assistants suggested they try agar, an extract of seaweed. Then an assistant devised a dish with a lid specially designed for culturing. His name was Robert Petri, and today the Petri dish is familiar to biology students everywhere.

Koch was also very important in developing procedures for staining bacteria. Some of these creatures were difficult, if not impossible, to observe under the microscope. Koch worked out ways of coloring them to make them more visible. This, too, was an important breakthrough in the study of microbes. Staining is now taught in high-school biology courses. Koch was learning how to manipulate bacteria. Eventually he identified and described the anthrax bacterium, which Pasteur built on to develop his vaccine.

With all the evidence that was piling up, it would seem that the germ theory was proven. But there were still many who were unconvinced about microbes, and the miasma theory was still accepted by many. And it remained true that disease seemed to strike in a random way that was hard to predict or account for otherwise.

It is important for us to remember that this period, around the middle of the nineteenth century, saw the Industrial Revolution reaching a

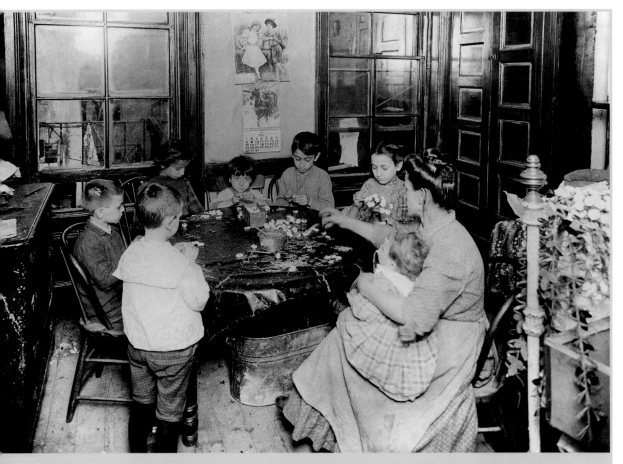

AS POPULATIONS GREW AND FARM WORK BECAME MORE AND MORE MECHANIZED, PEOPLE BEGAN CROWDING INTO THE CITIES. MANY FOUND FACTORY JOBS, BUT SOME, SUCH AS THIS WOMAN AND HER CHILDREN, WORKED AT HOME IN CROWDED APARTMENTS WHERE SEVERAL PEOPLE SHARED EACH BED. INFECTIOUS DISEASES SPREAD RAPIDLY IN SUCH CONDITIONS.

climax in America and western Europe. Put simply, beginning in England in the middle of the eighteenth century, new technologies were being developed for making products by machine that had previously been made at home by hand. Instead of spinning and weaving at home, housewives bought cloth made in factories. Improved agricultural machinery made it possible for fewer workers to produce more food. Many farmworkers, no longer needed, drifted into towns and cities. A better food supply helped to make populations grow. Towns grew into cities; cities began to spread out across the countryside, swallowing up forests

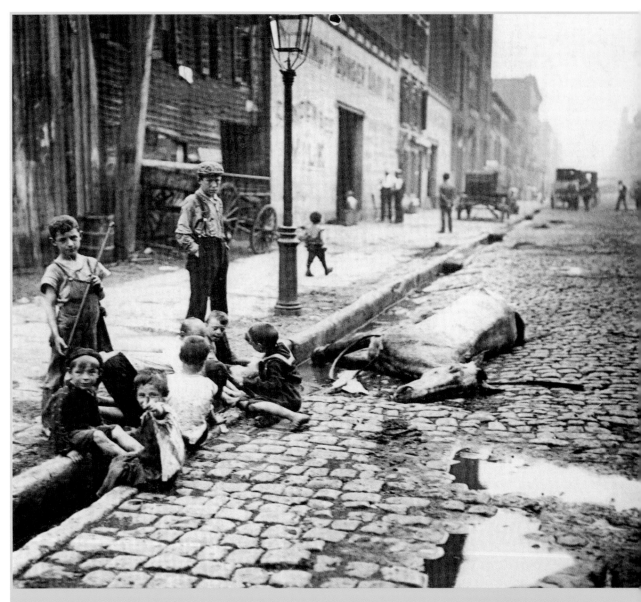

IF HOMES WERE UNSANITARY, STREETS WERE EVEN WORSE. HERE CHILDREN PLAY IN A GUTTER RUNNING WITH FILTHY WATER NEXT TO THE BODY OF A HORSE. DEATH RATES FROM INFECTIOUS DISEASES WERE ESPECIALLY HIGH IN CITIES.

and farmland. In a hundred years the population of major cities doubled and then tripled.

The growth of cities was uncontrolled. Factory owners wanted labor nearby; workers wanted jobs in factories. But there was not enough housing, clean water, or garbage- and sewage-disposal systems to take care of the increased amounts of human and animal waste. Sewage was sluiced into local rivers through open channels running down the middle of main streets. Garbage, even dead horses, sat in heaps for days before it was collected.

Water was often drawn from the same rivers into which sewage flowed, or at best from nearby wells, which were always at risk of contamination. Given what we know about sanitation today, it is hardly surprising that disease was everywhere, and epidemics were commonplace. But as long as the miasma theory of disease prevailed, there seemed no reason to clean up the streets except for cosmetic purposes.

It was the poor—and most working people were poor—who suffered. They lived in crowded conditions, often several people to a room and three or four people to a bed; disease was easily passed from one person to the next. Where more affluent citizens were able to have garbage and waste removed, working people lived surrounded by it. In those conditions people were often sick, some of them most of the time, and they routinely died of diseases we rarely even see today.

One such disease was tuberculosis. It is a disease of the lungs, although it can also affect the bones and other organs. In the nineteenth century it killed slowly but surely; victims might survive for years, in the end drowning in fluid in their lungs. It affected everybody—John Keats, one of the greatest English poets, died of it in his twenties—but it was especially a disease of the poor. During this time it was responsible for 15 percent of all deaths in Europe and America. As a killer it was far more deadly than other feared diseases such as rabies.

By 1880 Koch was beginning to be recognized as an important researcher, and the German government set up an advanced laboratory for him, with assistants and all the equipment he needed. Koch was expected to make significant advances in medicine, and he tackled tuberculosis. In 1882 he identified the tuberculosis bacterium. His attempts to find a vaccine failed; not until 1921 would an even partially successful tuberculosis vaccine be made. However, Koch's work showed that tuberculosis was transmitted from person to person through tiny droplets of moisture expelled into the air from tubercular lungs.

So even though he did not find a vaccine, Koch's work suggested ways to reduce the death toll. For one, it became customary to send tuberculosis victims to sanitoriums, especially in mountainous or desert areas where the air was likely to contain fewer bacteria. This not only isolated tuberculosis patients from others, but was thought to improve their chances for recovery. For another, cities mounted strong campaigns against spitting. Before that time spitting had been customary in many places. In the eighteenth century Americans routinely spit in church. By the nineteenth century there was a growing revulsion against spitting, but it was still customary in public places: spittoons were found in saloons, hotel lobbies, and railroad stations. Then laws were passed against spitting in public, and slowly spittoons disappeared. Finally, the war against tuberculosis added force to a general movement toward cleaning up cities, which began in the early part of the twentieth century.

The lesson that sanitation was crucial to good health was made all the more clear in the battle against yet another frightful disease we no long worry about in the industrial world, cholera. Some historians believe that the disease dates back to before the time of Christ; but if so, it was confined to a few regions of Asia. Not until the nineteenth century did it become a serious scourge in Europe and America. The disease causes violent vomiting and diarrhea, which in turn dehydrates the body. Then muscle spasms, circulatory collapse, and death can follow. Some 20 to 50 percent of cholera victims died, usually in a few days, but sometimes within hours.

Cholera began to spread from Asia in the early nineteenth century when the British overlords in India improved the local transportation system in order to speed the movement of goods and people, and thus advance trade. Roads, railways, and enlarged docking facilities were built. People began to travel more, both around India and back and forth between India and England. Inevitably some of them were bearing cholera.

An early cholera epidemic in the Caribbean had dramatic effects on the future of the United States. In about 1800 the French dictator Napoléon Bonaparte, who was trying to build an empire in the Caribbean, sent troops to stop a rebellion of slaves on the island of Santo Domingo, now Haiti and the Dominican Republic. A cholera epidemic swept through the French troops, claiming most of them. The rebellion succeeded and created the nation of Haiti, which former slaves took over and ruled. Shortly afterward Napoléon decided to give up on the Caribbean. France at the time claimed a huge portion of North America west of the Mississippi. Napoléon sold this land to President Thomas Jefferson. Known as the Louisiana Purchase, it doubled the area of the United States.

Through the nineteenth century there were several pandemics of cholera (the disease spread over a large geographic area); one began in 1817 and lasted until 1823. Through the nineteenth century millions died. Like tuberculosis, cholera was particularly a disease of the poor, but for some time the connection to sanitation was not made. Then, in the middle of the century, a London doctor named John Snow started mapping the city's cholera cases. He noticed a cluster of cases with a high death rate around Broad Street. He investigated and discovered that all the families in that area drew their water from the same pump. He persuaded city authorities to remove the handle from the pump. Suddenly the cases of cholera in Broad Street ended.

A similar instance occurred in Germany, in the city of Hamburg. A political division ran down the middle of one street. Water for both sides of the street was drawn from the Elbe River. However the water for one side of the street passed through a treatment plant, but for the other side it did not. On the side getting treated water, there was no cholera; on the other side, there was a wealth of cases. Instances such as Broad Street and Hamburg ought to have alerted people to the possible causes of the disease. Sometimes it did, but the miasma theory still hung on.

Then, in 1883, there was a severe outbreak of cholera in Egypt, across the Mediterranean from Europe, and there was considerable fear that the disease would spread. Pasteur and Koch were asked by their governments to see if they could discover the cause of cholera and, if possible, a cure. Pasteur was in poor health and couldn't make the trip, but sent a team; Koch himself headed the German team. As usual the antagonistic French and German groups were determined to beat each other to the cholera bacteria. In the end Koch and the Germans "won." Koch showed that the bacteria were swarming not only in the polluted water of overcrowded Egyptian cities, but in the food and elsewhere as well. Cholera was being recycled from the ill through sewage back into local water and then into other victims. Thus, even though Koch did not find a vaccine for cholera, he showed that proper sanitation, especially water treatment, could slow the spread of the disease. Gradually governments, mostly in Europe and America, began to improve the sanitation of their cities and towns.

By the 1880s the work of Pasteur, Koch, and other microbe hunters had been widely publicized. Pasteur in particular had become an international hero. Inevitably, ambitious young doctors and biologists began looking for the microbes responsible for others of the great array of diseases making life a misery for so many millions of humans. Any person who found a cure, or even the cause, of such diseases was certain to achieve fame as a great benefactor of humankind. So in labs across Europe, America, and elsewhere, young biologists got out their microscopes and set to work.

Another tragic disease besetting people at the time was diphtheria. It mainly afflicted children, their nerves slowly paralyzed by the toxin produced by the bacteria that caused the disease. A Frenchman and a

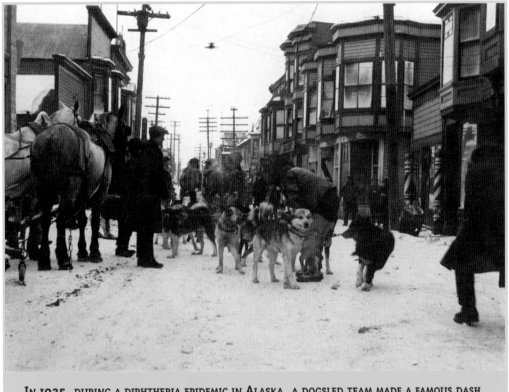

IN 1925, DURING A DIPHTHERIA EPIDEMIC IN ALASKA, A DOGSLED TEAM MADE A FAMOUS DASH TO THE TOWN OF NOME WITH A SUPPLY OF DIPHTHERIA ANTITOXIN. NEWSPAPERS CARRIED THE STORY ACROSS THE COUNTRY.

German, competing as always, began studying diphtheria. The Frenchman was Emile Roux, from the Pasteur Institute, and the German was Emil Behring, a disciple of Koch's. Working separately and then eventually together, they produced what is called an antitoxin, which significantly reduced the death rates from diphtheria. (A toxin is a poison. An antitoxin combats it.)

It is not possible in a book of this size to describe in detail how the body fights off infectious diseases, and even less how infectious diseases work. But we need to understand these processes at least in a rough way.

The body has three lines of defense against pathogens—that is, disease-causing foreign bodies such as viruses, bacteria, fungi, and toxins.

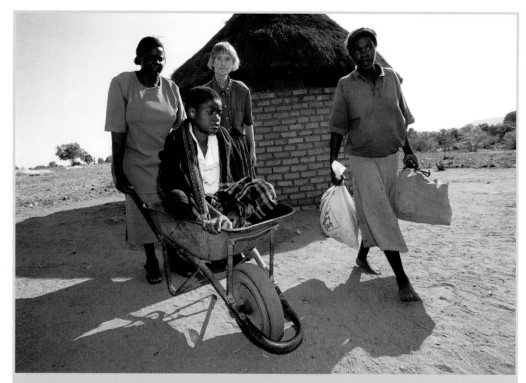

THE SCOURGE OF TUBERCULOSIS LINGERS IN DEVELOPING NATIONS. THIS 2001 PHOTOGRAPH SHOWS A TUBERCULOSIS PATIENT BEING WHEELED TO A CAR THAT WILL TAKE HER TO A HOSPITAL. IN UNSANITARY CONDITIONS, TUBERCULOSIS SPREADS EASILY.

The first line of defense is the body's surface, essentially the skin, which prevents pathogens from entering, unless it is broken from a cut or a splinter. Skin also secretes certain chemicals that help to destroy pathogens.

The second line of defense is inflammation, the swelling that appears when we get a bruise or a cut. Inflammation is a complicated response, involving a variety of body cells, which helps to repair damage, neutralize toxins, and prevent the spread of microbial invaders.

The third line of defense is the immune system. This is a very complex reaction, and even today it has not been entirely understood. In simple terms, certain of the cells normally present in the blood are primed to recognize foreign invaders such as viruses and bacteria. These are mainly white blood cells called lymphocytes, although other cells are involved as well. Once the white blood cells recognize the presence of invaders, they trigger a chain of events that in the end produces what are called antibodies—chemical molecules that attach themselves to the invaders and destroy them.

But there is more to it than that. Once antibodies have been produced to fight off a certain type of invader, special cells maintain a "memory" of that invader. When that invader appears next it will immediately begin producing antibodies. This is how—once again, roughly speaking—vaccines work. They introduce invaders in a form mild enough not to endanger the body, but strong enough to encourage the production of antibodies. The cells "remember"—and when a real invader strikes, they go to work producing the right kind of antibodies to repel it. It is a little like a war game, in which soldiers practice war against a pretend enemy so they will learn how to respond when facing a real one.

The body has to produce a special antibody to fight each specific pathogen it encounters. Antibodies for smallpox, for example, are no use against cholera. Although in a few rare cases an antibody for one pathogen will also fight a second one, generally there is a specific antibody for each pathogen.

This is the reason why researchers have had to find so many different types of vaccines—one for each pathogen. And it also will explain why in certain instances, like influenza, it has been difficult to come up with a permanent vaccine for the disease. We think of influenza, or *flu* as we usually say, as a bothersome but harmless illness that strikes us occasionally in the winter, causing us to miss a day or so of school or work, and then passes. It is not: the influenza epidemic that swept the world in 1918 was one of the worst killers humanity has ever seen.

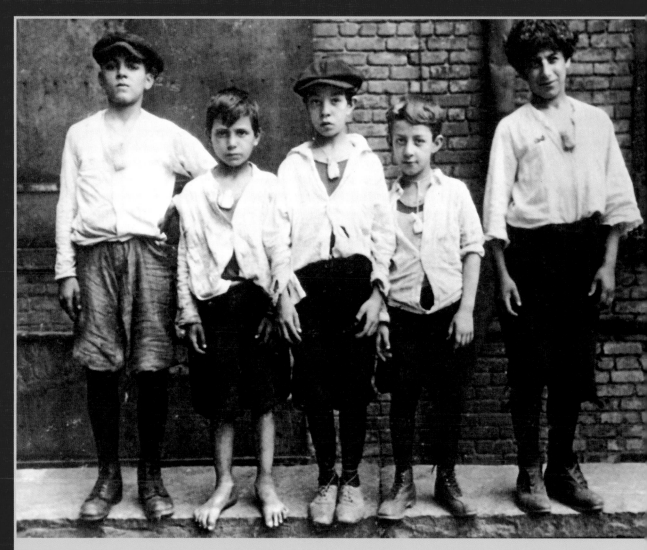

WHEN THE INFLUENZA EPIDEMIC OF 1918 STRUCK, SCIENTISTS KNEW THAT VIRUSES, AS THEY WERE CALLED, EXISTED, BUT THEY COULD NOT DETECT THEM IN THE MICROSCOPES OF THE TIME. THUS THEY DID NOT UNDERSTAND HOW VIRUSES FUNCTIONED OR HOW THEY COULD BE DEFEATED. AS A RESULT, MANY DIFFERENT FOLK REMEDIES WERE TRIED. THESE BOYS ARE WEARING BAGS OF CAMPHOR AROUND THEIR NECKS, WHICH OF COURSE PROVED USELESS AGAINST A VIRUS.

The Forgotten Plague

The great influenza pandemic of 1918 is a mystery within a mystery. To this day scientists are not sure how it started or where it came from, although theories abound. More mysterious is the fact that the epidemic has almost wholly dropped out of human awareness. It is virtually never spoken of anymore. It has been a long time since any of us has ever heard an old man or woman tell stories of the bodies stacked up along the roads to cemeteries because there were not enough people available to bury them, the great battles of World War I called off because the soldiers were too sick to fight. This epidemic did not take place in the Middle Ages, or even in the grimy, garbage-littered streets of Victorian London. It took place in America, along with the rest of the world, so recently that most Americans in their nineties are old enough to have experienced it—to have even flirted with death themselves during it. But they never speak of it. Nor, if you look in history books, will you find much about it besides a passing reference in a sentence or two.

Yet within a few months, the influenza epidemic of 1918 killed at least 40 million people worldwide, and some responsible authorities think the number may have been as high as 100 million. By comparison World War I, which was winding down at the time of the epidemic, killed about 10 million men. No other event in human history, no plague or war, has killed so many people in so short a time.

World War I began in Europe in 1914. Americans tried to stay out of it, but in 1917 they were drawn in, although not until early in 1918 were large numbers of American soldiers actually fighting. To some extent the war acted as a catalyst for influenza because it meant that millions of people, mostly soldiers, were being packed together in training camps, barracks, ships, and trenches. Millions of others were being shifted around Europe or being sent from various parts of the world to fight in France. Inevitably wartime conditions helped to spread the disease.

The influenza epidemic was prefaced by a mild and brief epidemic of the disease in the spring of 1918. It was first noticed in Spain and, as a consequence, got the name Spanish flu, which is still often used, although there is no evidence that the disease actually originated in Spain. By summer this brief siege had died out.

In August 1918 navy vessels were constantly passing in and out of American harbors. On August 28, eight sailors in Boston got sick with the flu. Nobody was particularly worried. But the next day more sailors were sick, and then more. Then civilians in Boston began to catch the disease too. Boston's hospitals filled up, and within days the patients were dying.

The disease then spread to Camp Devens, near Boston. There were 50,000 men in the camp, and within a few weeks so many of the soldiers were sick that the usual military training and drills had to be canceled. Special trains were hired to take away the corpses, and many bodies were simply stacked up in empty barracks to await burial.

The Spanish flu of 1918 attacked the lungs—it was eventually discovered that it could live only in the warm, moist environment of lung tissue. As the flu destroyed the lungs, the body grew starved for oxygen. The extremities, such as the feet and ears, turned black from lack of oxygen, and the blackness spread across the face. By then the lungs were being damaged, filling up with fluid. The victim gasped for breath, bloody spittle forming at the mouth. For hours, or possibly days, the victim choked to death in agony. In some cases the disease would kill in less than a day: one doctor saw a soldier walking across a parade ground simply fall down dead as he walked.

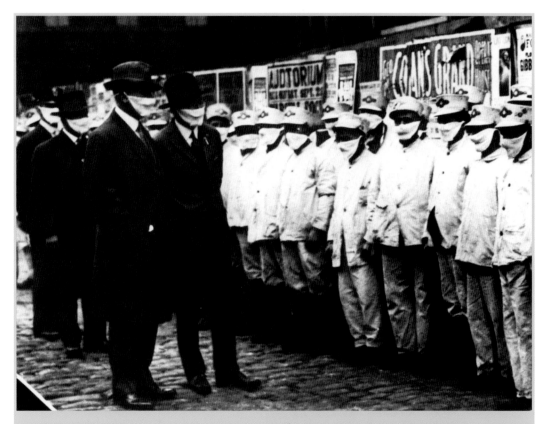

THE MASKS WORN BY THESE OFFICIALS INSPECTING CHICAGO SANITATION WORKERS WERE OF LITTLE HELP IN SHIELDING THEM FROM THE FLU VIRUS. BUT PEOPLE, SEEING DEATH ALL AROUND THEM, WERE DESPERATE FOR ANYTHING THAT MIGHT SPARE THEM.

By October the disease was everywhere in the United States and was appearing simultaneously in Europe, Asia, and Africa. Practically no area was exempt. The flu seemed to have sprung out of nowhere in a thousand places at once. Even today, investigators are not able to explain adequately how the disease appeared in so many distant places simultaneously.

And there was no cure. It was caused by a virus, not a bacterium—that much was known. But at that time nobody really knew what a virus was. However, as pathologists couldn't find bacteria in affected tissues, by a process of elimination they had to assume that the flu was caused by a virus.

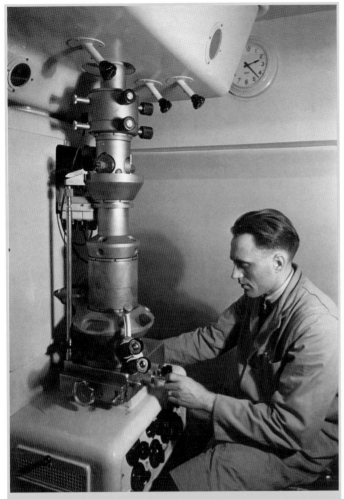

THIS 1950 PHOTOGRAPH SHOWS A SCIENTIST USING AN ELECTRON MICROSCOPE IN HIS LABORATORY AT MILL HILL IN LONDON, ENGLAND, WHERE MAJOR RESEARCH ON THE INFLUENZA VIRUS WAS CONDUCTED.

Then, in 1934, the electron microscope was invented. Eventually it was capable of revealing much smaller bits of matter than the regular light microscope could. By the late 1940s viruses could be seen. What they were made of was another matter. Not until the 1950s, when the discovery of the DNA double helix allowed the deciphering of the genetic code, was it learned that viruses were short bits of either DNA or RNA surrounded by protein. They are merely short strings of genes, and the question remains whether or not they ought to be considered living matter. For one thing, bacteria can reproduce as cells do, by dividing. Viruses cannot reproduce on their own. Yet on the other hand, as we will see, they evolve, as most living things do. It is a hard question to answer.

In any case viruses replicate, or make copies of themselves, only by penetrating one of the billions of cells that make up a living body, and using the machinery inside the cell to duplicate themselves, sometimes in vast numbers. The cell is destroyed in this process, although not necessarily immediately, as the many viruses escape to infect other cells, where they produce more copies and destroy those cells too.

Clearly this process can take place very rapidly: a single virus can produce several thousand copies of itself in a few hours; each one of those new viruses can infect a cell and proceed to produce thousands of more copies in another few hours. A little multiplication shows that in the course of a day one virus can turn into millions, and in another day those millions of viruses can become trillions.

Viruses, thus, can be extremely destructive. Why is it that they have not long since destroyed the human race? For one thing, most viruses are to one extent or another selective: as we have seen, the flu viruses can live only in the moist, warm atmosphere of the lungs and will not harm other organs of the body. If the lungs survive the viral attack, the patient will live. For another, there are those antibodies that very quickly attack invading viruses. It is true that antibodies cannot penetrate cells to kill viruses already lodged there, but antibodies can catch viruses when they are circulating between cells. And in many cases the patient who survives a viral attack will develop an immunity to that virus for the future.

But there is another, more subtle reason why microbes, both bacteria and viruses, don't always kill their hosts. No form of life can afford to wipe out its source of essential supplies. In simple terms farmers must always save some of the corn they grow to provide seed for next year's crop. So corn goes on existing because farmers can't afford to eat all of it at once. Likewise a virus cannot afford to wipe out its hosts. Only microbes that leave some people (or animals) alive are likely to last over time.

The influenza virus of 1918 affected a quarter of the American people. Among the people confined together in large numbers, the rates were much higher: 40 percent of the men in the navy and 36 percent of the ground soldiers suffered from influenza. The flu killed 2.5 percent of them. That may seem like a small number, but it translated into hundreds of thousands of deaths. If we apply the same numbers to the American population today it would come out to 1.5 million people—more Americans than have died in all our wars combined.

In 1918 it was enough to throw Americans—indeed people everywhere—into a panic. In the Philadelphia morgue the bodies were piled three deep "in the corridors and in almost every room." Some undertakers refused to bury the dead and forced the relatives to dig the graves. People began wearing gauze masks in the streets; places such as Tucson, Arizona, required masks to be worn in public. In many cities and towns, schools, movie theaters, and dance halls were closed. In Streator, Illinois, the dead were lined up along the road, waiting their turn to be buried. In France the Eighty-eighth Division fought on the front lines from mid-September to late October: 90 of them were killed, wounded, or captured; 444 died of the flu. The death rate among soldiers was so high that one German general believed that the influenza would wipe out the French army and save the Germans from defeat. In the United States the army suspended the draft, quarantined army camps, and reduced the amount of training. In Washington, D.C., the Supreme Court shut down to save lawyers—and no doubt themselves—from catching the disease in what was usually a crowded courtroom. Incredibly some towns made it a crime to sneeze in public. In New York huge steam shovels were used to dig mass graves. And everywhere, when a family member fell ill, there was panic.

The disease was completely unpredictable: some died in two or three days; others recovered in the same amount of time. And then, as suddenly as it had come, the great influenza pandemic dwindled and died out. But its effects were so great in the course of a few weeks that the life expectancy for 1918 in the United States dropped twelve years from what it had been the year before.

So the epidemic came and went, and still nobody knew what had caused it or how the disease could be cured. You would think that a massive effort would have been mounted to find a cure, a vaccine, at least the cause, to prevent the disease's return. It appeared that nobody wanted to think about it; the dreadful scourge was better forgotten. So the great influenza pandemic slipped from the collective memory and did not make it into the history textbooks we use today.

Fortunately there were a few who remembered. One of them was Richard E. Shope, who grew up on an Iowa farm, became a doctor, and then turned to medical research. He got a job at the Rockefeller Institute, a famous medical research center in New York City. Shope and others had noticed that in 1918, at the time of the flu epidemic, there had also been an epidemic of swine flu. Shope set about experimenting with hogs. At first he tried to find a bacterium for swine flu, but could not, and then went in search of a virus. He could not find that either.

In England, however, some other scientists were also struggling with the problem of human flu. They had, of course, to experiment with animals, and the problem was, as always, to find an animal that was susceptible to the human disease. They discovered that ferrets—small, sometimes very fierce animals that originally had been bred to chase rats and rabbits out of their holes—could catch the flu. Shope and the British combined forces. They soon realized that swine flu and human flu were, if not identical, related. Among other things, people who had been alive during the 1918 epidemic often developed antibodies that would block swine flu. But unfortunately there was still nothing known that could attack human flu viruses.

There were, however, plenty of cases of flu around. Nothing like the 1918 epidemic occurred, but waves of flu continued to make regular appearances—about eleven years apart, it seemed to some investigators. These waves were not harmless: each one killed tens of thousands of Americans.

So the scientists kept working. An important breakthrough came in 1936, when it was learned that the flu viruses could be grown in fertilized eggs. When you work with pathogens, you need a lot of samples. The use of fertilized eggs as a medium in which to grow the flu viruses was immensely helpful. Eggs were much cheaper than experimental animals such as ferrets, and it was far easier to inoculate an egg with a virus than to give a shot to an angry, snarling ferret. Once inside the egg membrane, the embryo would draw the virus into its lung tissue, where it would rapidly grow in the usual way and then spill back into the surrounding fluid—the egg white.

With the use of the electron microscope, it was soon discovered that there were basically two types of flu virus. One was called type A, and this was the class of viruses that humans were most likely to contract. Humans could also get type B, but it was less frequent. Most important for our understanding of flu, scientists learned that type A flu viruses were genetically unstable: they could easily change in some small but significant way, turning into a new strain.

In some cases new strains of influenza emerged when two different flu viruses ended up inside the same cell in a given host. This occasionally happened in swine, which could harbor both human and swine flu. In this circumstance different flu viruses could exchange genetic material, creating a third type of virus different enough to withstand antibodies designed to destroy the strains of viruses it came from.

More commonly viruses change through the normal mechanism of evolution. Evolution is a complex process, the details of which are still argued about by biologists. To put it simply, in the case of viruses, sometimes the strings of genetic material that make up a virus are imperfectly copied in the host cell. The new virus, then, is slightly different from its parent strain. In most cases these small changes, or mutations, are meaningless. However occasionally a mutation will produce a new virus that is able to elude antibodies, and this can be particularly dangerous. As it happens, viral RNA, which the flu virus consists of, is particularly unstable. As a consequence new strains of flu are frequently produced. Given the speed with which viruses can reproduce in their host cells, these new versions of the flu virus can spread rapidly.

By the late 1930s researchers had learned a good deal about how the flu virus works. In 1944 a vaccine was developed that would immunize against influenza. This vaccine was a so-called killed virus, in which the virus was dead, as opposed to the attenuated type Pasteur had used for his vaccines. A killed virus cannot cause the disease at all, but the immune system will react to it as if the virus were alive, and start producing antibodies.

The flu vaccine would work only against one particular strain of flu. In order to truly protect people against flu, it would be necessary to create an array of vaccines to match dozens of flu strains, including some that had yet to develop.

That is how the situation remains today. It now appears that between human outbreaks, flu viruses reside in animal reservoirs. Researchers believe that the primary reservoir for flu is domestic fowl living in the southern part of China. Here ducks and pigs are raised together in wet rice fields. In a situa-

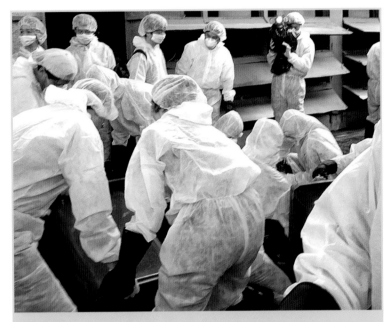

HONG KONG WORKERS REMOVE DEAD CHICKENS FROM GARBAGE BINS IN AN EFFORT TO PREVENT THE SPREAD OF BIRD FLU IN MAY 2001. PROMPT ACTION HALTED WHAT MIGHT HAVE BEEN A SIGNIFICANT FLU EPIDEMIC.

tion such as this, there are endless opportunities for different strains of virus to mingle in their animal hosts. Inevitably from time to time a new strain, deadly to humans, breaks out.

This happened in 1997 in Hong Kong, which shares a border with the province of Guangdong in southern China. The first-known victim was a three-year-old boy who became suddenly ill and soon died. The Hong Kong health officials were alarmed, for they had a killer disease on their hands and no idea where it was coming from.

Among other places, they turned to the Center for Disease Control and Prevention (CDC) in Atlanta, Georgia, an arm of the U.S. government, which is considered one of the most advanced institutions of its kind in the world. The CDC, among its many roles, is supposed to determine the causes of new infectious diseases wherever they break out. It is a vital outpost in not merely America's but the world's front-line defense against disease. The CDC quickly identified the new virus as a bird virus, which should not have affected humans. Perhaps the death of the three-year-old boy was a fluke, an isolated case.

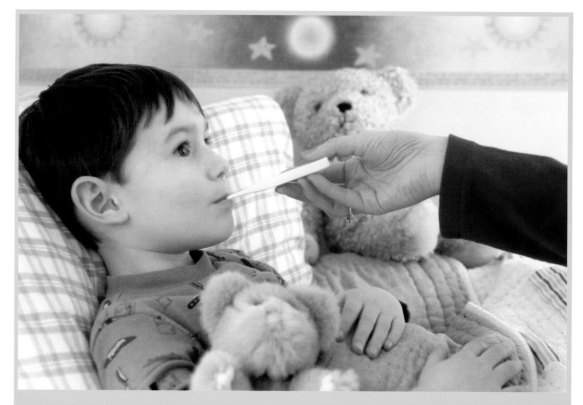

INFLUENZA HAS BY NO MEANS BEEN DEFEATED. COUNTLESS PEOPLE STILL CONTRACT IT EVERY YEAR, AND FOR SOME IT STILL LEADS TO DEATH.

But it was not. Humans were getting the disease. By that winter there were eighteen more cases, eight very serious ones resulting in six deaths. Where was the disease coming from? The best guess was chickens. Hong Kong is heavily populated, and there is only limited space for farms. Much of the food comes from mainland China, including 80 percent of the chickens. Researchers from the CDC, the Hong Kong health authority, and elsewhere went to work and soon identified the cause as chickens imported to Hong Kong from China. Hong Kong authorities ordered the slaughter of a million live chickens already in Hong Kong poultry markets. New birds coming in would be quarantined until it was certain that they were not ill, and random testing of chickens would be performed. The epidemic of what is now known as the Hong Kong flu was stopped in time.

But the danger had been very real. Millions of tourists, students, and businesspeople from all over the world pass through Hong Kong every year. Citizens of Hong Kong routinely visit China, Taiwan, Japan, Korea, and other places around Asia, and many of them come to the Americas on business or to visit relatives. If the disease had not been so rapidly contained, largely because of quick cooperation among the various health authorities, the world might have seen yet another flu pandemic like the Spanish flu, with deaths running into the tens of millions.

Nor is the danger over. Recently a group of so-called plug drugs has been developed, which fill a cavity in a flu virus where it clings to its host and prevents the virus's harmful effects. The problem with the plug drugs is that you often have a virus for several days before you know what you are sick with, and by then the disease may have progressed too far for plug drugs to be effective.

At the moment the most effective preventive measure remains flu shots. At the beginning of each year, influenza experts under the auspices of international health bodies decide which strain of flu is likely to be most dangerous during the following winter. A vaccine is quickly produced and in the fall is made available to doctors. Currently it is generally advised that older people, who are most likely to die from the disease, have the new flu shot each fall. The vaccines provide only about 80 percent immunity, but they certainly reduce the chances of death from flu.

Unfortunately only the people who live in industrialized nations are usually able to afford flu shots. Most of the world's people go without, and experts today expect that sooner or later the world will see another influenza pandemic like the one in 1918. Given the fact that there are vastly more people today than there were in 1918, the death toll could run to 100 million and perhaps even a great many more.

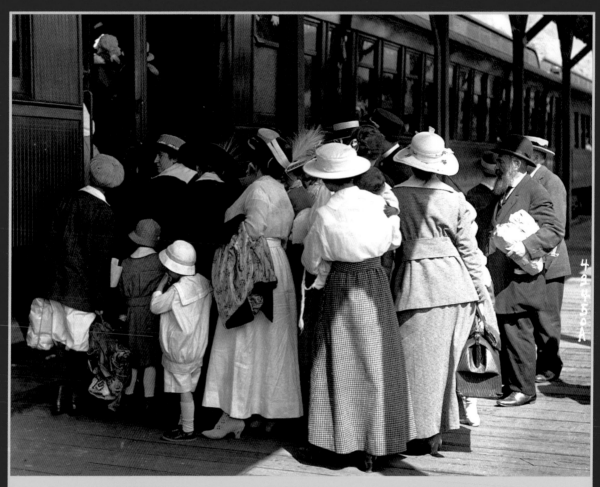

POLIO, OR INFANTILE PARALYSIS AS IT WAS THEN KNOWN, BROUGHT MISERY AND EVEN DEATH, ESPECIALLY TO CHILDREN. HERE, DURING A 1916 EPIDEMIC, PANICKED PARENTS BOARD A TRAIN WITH THEIR CHILDREN TO ESCAPE THE DANGERS OF THE CITY.

The Great Crippler

There are many infectious diseases that cause suffering around the world. Vaccines have been developed for some of these, but not for all. Still among the worst killers are hemophilus influenza, causing 3.7 million deaths annually; tuberculosis, 2.9 million deaths even though there is a vaccine available; cholera, 2.5 million deaths; and the new killer, AIDS, which currently causes 2.3 million deaths, with the rate certain to go up.

Still for Americans, there is no doubt that the most dramatic story in the struggle against disease was the race for the polio vaccine. Polio existed in other countries, but the United States was particularly hard hit. We have seen how increased efforts were made to clean up cities, when medical researchers finally began to understand that infectious diseases were caused by microbes that could live in water, garbage, and sewage. This was especially true in the United States. In the early part of the twentieth century, President Theodore Roosevelt championed a social and political movement called the Progressive movement. One of the important goals of the Progressive movement was to clean up America's cities, which were teeming with poor, often ill-educated immigrants, many of whom had come from farms and were unaccustomed to city life. The Progressive notion was to write laws requiring less crowded dwellings with more sun and air, cleaner water, milk and other foods, and better sanitation. The Progressive movement by no means eliminated poverty and dirt, but it did make significant progress in improving waste disposal and water supplies. Cities became healthier and, paradoxically, that led to an upsurge of infantile paralysis, or poliomyelitis, to use the current name.

The reason was simple: previously children living in the old, unsanitary slums were exposed to a lot of different infections; many of the children died, but the ones who lived acquired immunity to many diseases. In the cleaner cities children were exposed to fewer diseases and had less natural immunity to them. When such diseases struck, they struck hard. One such disease was polio.

The disease had existed for thousands of years; evidence for it can be found in the bones of people who died in ancient times. But it had never been a major fear. By the middle of the nineteenth century, there began to be occasional small outbreaks of the disease. Not much was known about it, except that autopsies of victims showed inflammation of part of the spinal cord. Mild cases often went undetected. It has been estimated that by 1880 perhaps 1 percent of the cases led to paralysis.

The first big outbreak in the United States came in 1916, not surprisingly about a generation after the Progressive movement began its work. It appears to have begun in New York City, although it is always difficult to be sure where a disease first appears. From there it moved into New York's suburbs, where an even cleaner environment had left children with even less immunity to infectious diseases.

A polio victim generally suffered first from a cold, then a headache, then chills. Within a few days some kind of paralysis would set in. The paralysis might be mild, amounting to nothing more than a stiff joint, which would clear up, leaving the sufferer perfectly healthy. But the paralysis could be severe, likely to affect the legs, but it could extend to other parts of the body too. In the worst cases virtually the whole body became paralyzed, which meant that the victim could no longer move the muscles of the upper torso in order to breathe. These people, many of them little children, would lie in their beds gasping for breath hour after hour, day after day. Sometimes they would improve; but in the severest cases the victims would be left permanently disabled, unable to use their legs and perhaps a hand or arm.

In the 1916 epidemic there were 27,000 cases across 26 states. Undoubtedly there were many more mild cases that went undetected. Six thousand died; thousands were left crippled. Many ended up living in iron lungs, body-length chambers that helped the victim to breathe.

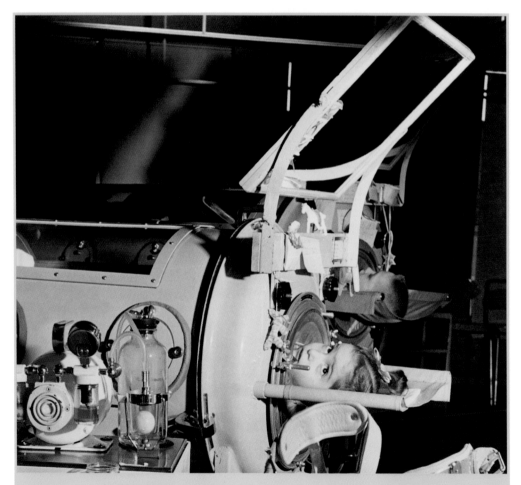

SOMETIMES POLIO PARALYZED CHILDREN FROM THE NECK DOWN, LEAVING THEM UNABLE TO BREATHE ON THEIR OWN. THESE CHILDREN LIVED IN IRON LUNGS. SOME OF THEM REMAINED IN THEM FOR THE DURATION OF THEIR LIVES.

Others were confined to wheelchairs for life or were left with one or more useless limbs.

For a while after the outbreak, the disease rates dropped somewhat, but then they began to climb again through the 1930s and into the 1940s. In 1948 there were again 27,000 cases; in 1950 there were 33,000; and in 1952 there were 59,000. The United States was the world center for polio.

And there was no cure. As its early name, infantile paralysis, suggests, at first it was mainly a disease of children; but it struck older people too. Despite polio's penchant for striking children, its most famous victim was an adult, Franklin D. Roosevelt. In 1921, at age 39, Roosevelt had already been an assistant secretary to the Navy and in 1920 a candidate for the vice presidency. Although his ticket had lost, he was considered a great political prospect. Charming, handsome, well-educated, and confident, Roosevelt had bright prospects. Then he was struck down by polio, which left his legs paralyzed. For seven years, through exercise and anything else he could think of, he tried to walk again. He never succeeded. For the rest of his life he was able to stand only for short periods by locking his leg braces, usually holding on to something for support.

Among other attempts to improve his mobility, he began visiting what was then a run-down resort in Warm Springs, Georgia. Swimming in the hot pool there was supposed to help polio victims. It didn't, but swimming did improve the strength in Roosevelt's arms, which helped him to get around better on crutches.

Roosevelt went back into politics. In 1928 he became governor of New York State, and in 1932 he was elected president. He would win three more terms, to be the longest serving of all American presidents. During the Depression of the 1930s, he set in motion great changes in the U.S. government, among other things introducing Social Security. He went on to lead the United States to victory in World War II. His suffering from polio is thought to have made him sympathetic to the plight

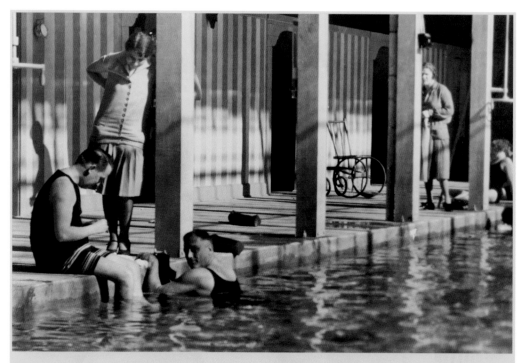

THE MOST FAMOUS VICTIM OF POLIO WAS FRANKLIN D. ROOSEVELT (THIRD FROM LEFT), WHO LATER BECAME ONE OF AMERICA'S MOST ADMIRED PRESIDENTS. HERE HE SWIMS IN A POOL IN THE WARM SPRINGS, GEORGIA, RESORT HE TURNED INTO A CENTER FOR POLIO VICTIMS.

of the underprivileged in American society, leading to legislation such as unemployment insurance to aid those in need.

In the 1920s Roosevelt had bought the Warm Springs resort, refurbished it, and made it a center for polio victims. When he became governor of New York, he asked a friend of his, Basil O'Connor, to take over the management of Warm Springs. O'Connor was a tough man who liked to have his way. One person who knew him later said, "O'Connor had an expectation that when he spoke he would be obeyed."

O'Connor was always looking for ways to support Warm Springs. He started holding special "birthday balls" on President Roosevelt's birthday, to which he would invite celebrities for publicity's sake. In 1938 one of these celebrities, a song-and-dance man named Eddie Cantor, suggested that O'Connor start a national fund-raising program to aid

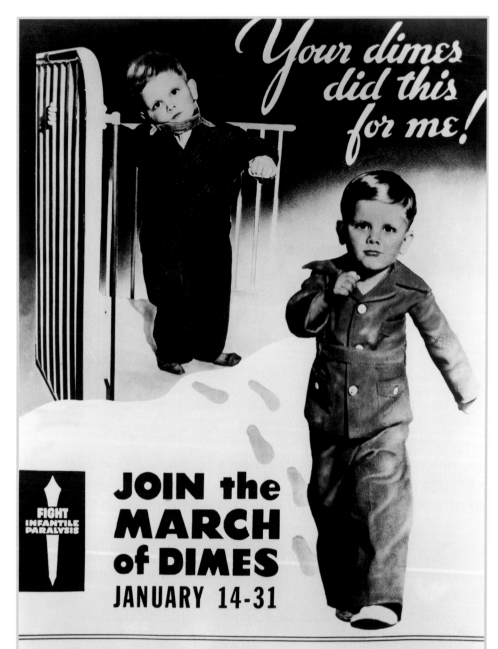

THE MARCH OF DIMES IS AN ENORMOUSLY SUCCESSFUL FUND-RAISING INSTITUTION. IT RAISED MUCH OF THE MONEY NEEDED FOR POLIO RESEARCH. IT INITIATED THE CONCEPT OF THE POSTER CHILD, AND EACH YEAR A NEW ONE WAS CHOSEN FOR THE FUND-RAISING CAMPAIGN.

the fight against polio. This became the March of Dimes, which is still in operation today.

The response to the idea was overwhelming for several reasons. For one, Americans, especially the parents of younger children, were thoroughly frightened of polio. The disease always seemed to strike hardest during the summer. Through the 1930s into the 1950s, families living in cities or nearby suburbs tried to send their children away to summer camps or to friends and relatives living in the country. Parents and grandparents of many of today's students can remember going off to the country year after year in their youths.

Adding to public concern was the fact that most polio victims did not die. Instead they were visible everywhere in braces, on crutches, or in wheelchairs. Churches, schools, as well as Boy and Girl Scout troops had polio victims among their members, a constant reminder of what the dreaded disease could do.

Finally, the affliction of President Roosevelt was in the back of people's minds. Not every American admired Roosevelt, but the majority did, and many idolized him. If Roosevelt asked them to join the war on polio, they would do it.

The March of Dimes was a tremendous success. Hollywood stars such as Bing Crosby and later Elvis Presley helped with the publicity. Every year a national polio poster child was chosen; many localities chose their own poster children as well. Whole cities got involved. San Diego invented a widely imitated porch-light campaign: on certain evenings home owners left their porch lights on, signaling that they had money to give to the March of Dimes. The polio campaign, with its poster children, celebrity supporters, and tens of thousands of volunteers, set the style for many similar fund-raising drives for charitable causes that go on today.

Through these efforts O'Connor's organization, the National Foundation for Infantile Paralysis, gathered a tremendous amount of money. This was not a government group, but a private one. O'Connor had effective control of how the money was spent. A great deal of it went, of course, to provide crutches, wheelchairs, iron lungs, and hospital facilities for polio victims. But a lot of it went into the search for a cure.

The cure remained elusive. As early as the nineteenth century, a German orthopedist named Jacob Heine had made some clinical studies of polio. In 1905 Oskar Medin, a Swedish researcher, figured out that the disease was infectious. Gradually the understanding of polio grew: it was learned that it was spread by personal contact, and that it would infect monkeys, which meant that they could be used as experimental animals.

In 1935 Dr. John Kolmer thought he had come up with a vaccine, based on an attenuated strain of the virus drawn from the spinal column of an infected monkey. Unfortunately, some of the children inoculated with the Kolmer vaccine became ill, and a few of them died. The vaccine was dropped. Another doctor, Maurice Brodie, tried using a killed virus. This proved to be safer than Kolmer's attenuated virus, but was not very effective.

Then, ironically, in 1950 Basil O'Connor's daughter Bettyann, a mother of five children, got polio and ended up in a wheelchair. Polio became the passion of O'Connor's life.

All the time, knowledge continued to advance. Previously it had been thought that the polio virus entered the body through the nose. By the late 1940s, however, it was understood that it entered through the mouth and went into the digestive system. It was communicated, as a rule, by intestinal waste, and could be spread, for example, by people who had not washed their hands after going to the toilet, at beaches, or because of the disposal of sewage in rivers where people might swim. Once in the body the virus moved in the bloodstream to the brain or spinal cord, where it attacked certain cells that send messages to the muscles. The muscles became paralyzed because the brain was no longer able to tell them what to do.

An important breakthrough came in 1948 when a team led by John

Enders learned how to grow the polio virus in the lab. This meant that it was no longer necessary to grow it in monkeys, which was an expensive and time-consuming process. With an ample supply of the virus to work with, several labs began studying it. It was soon discovered that there was not just one but three strains or types of polio virus, which was the reason the early vaccines of Kolmer and Brodie had not worked.

By 1950 the belief was growing that a vaccine for polio could be found. Indeed many people hoped that the discovery was imminent. One reason was that there was plenty of money available for research. Another was that scientists realized that anyone who found a polio vaccine would be celebrated as a great benefactor of humankind, as turned out to be the case.

One man driven to find the vaccine was Jonas Salk. He had started his career working at the University of Michigan under Thomas Francis, a well-known immunologist who was concentrating on flu. In 1947 Salk, still a young man, had been invited to the University of Pittsburgh Medical Center, where he was given the freedom to research what he wanted. He was soon asked to help with "typing" polio viruses—that is, identifying various strains—and this led him into polio research.

His mentor at the University of Michigan, Thomas Francis, had worked with killed viruses in his search for a flu vaccine. Salk decided to take the same route in his polio work: killed vaccines were safer. Another man, however, had a different idea. That was Albert Sabin. Sabin had gotten into polio research during World War II, when the government had sent him to Africa to investigate an outbreak of polio among American soldiers stationed there. He discovered that the local people living in that particular area were carriers of polio, but were immune to it, because they had been exposed as children. American soldiers, coming from more sanitary towns and cities, had not been exposed to polio and were easy victims.

When the war was over, Sabin decided to go on with his polio work. He chose to hunt for an attenuated virus. For one, attenuated viruses

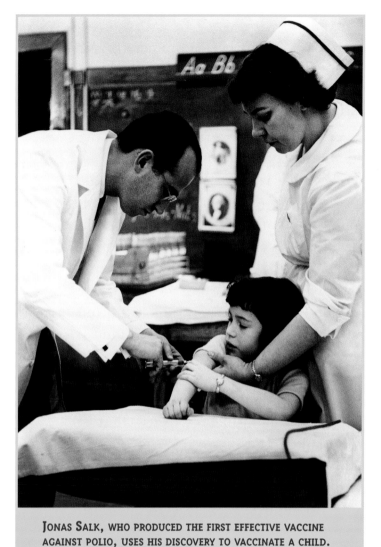

JONAS SALK, WHO PRODUCED THE FIRST EFFECTIVE VACCINE AGAINST POLIO, USES HIS DISCOVERY TO VACCINATE A CHILD.

were generally thought to be more effective than killed ones because they were more likely to trigger a strong immune response. For another, because people vaccinated with an attenuated virus got a mild form of the disease, they might pass it on to people they came in contact with, who would then become immune, as if they had had the shot themselves. Salk and Sabin of course knew of each other's work and, regrettably, they became competitors and eventually bitter rivals.

A killed virus, for technical reasons, could be developed faster, and Salk was the first to achieve it. By 1952 he was ready to conduct tests. This was a frightening moment, but one that could not be avoided if the vaccine was to be used. Amazingly the U.S. government had relatively little to do with what was going on. The program was still under the control of Basil O'Connor, who held the purse strings. He decided what experiments and what tests were done, because he chose which ones would get funded. Salk, according to his wife, Donna, had been willing to defer to O'Connor, and worked well with him. So Salk set out to do the first tests of his vaccine. He went to a place called the D. T. Watson Home, which housed a number of children who had suffered from the disease. As they had already had polio, they could not get it again. Salk, however, wanted to see if the vaccine would increase their immunity to it. The kids at Watson were scared of the shots, and some began crying. One of the attendants there, named Bill Kirkpatrick, volunteered to get a shot to show the children there was nothing for them to worry about. Kirkpatrick thus became the first human being to receive the Salk polio vaccine.

The trial at the Watson Home was successful. Salk next went to another home where the children had lived since infancy and so had not been exposed to polio or developed an immunity to it. Here too the trials were successful. Salk was now confident that his vaccine was safe and that it worked. He gave it to his own family and then to his lab assistants, none of whom could have been used as test subjects because they might well have acquired an immunity to polio through working with the virus.

By this time Salk and Sabin were barely speaking to each other. Sabin was telling people that Salk's vaccine might act as a booster, but wouldn't provide long-term immunity to polio. Making matters worse, Walter Winchell, a very influential newspaper columnist of the time, was spreading the story that the Salk vaccine was not safe and that O'Connor's organization was stockpiling thousands of coffins, a story that was untrue.

Nonetheless it was now time to go ahead with large-scale field trials of the vaccine. It was O'Connor's decision to move forward. He was exceedingly nervous about permitting the trials, which his organization would have to pay for. But there really was no choice, and in 1954 he authorized the trials to begin.

Thomas Francis, Salk's old mentor, was put in charge. Francis insisted on the most rigid specifications. He also insisted that nobody—not even Salk or O'Connor—would see the results of the trials until he had analyzed them himself and was willing to release them.

Surprisingly, despite the attacks on the Salk vaccine, particularly those by Winchell, more people volunteered to take the trial vaccine than could be used. Fear of polio was so great that parents everywhere wanted their children to participate. In the spring and summer of 1954, a mammoth test was conducted. Twenty thousand doctors, 40,000 nurses, 50,000 teachers, and 200,000 other volunteers helped to test 1.8 million children. No trial so massive had ever been attempted in the United States, and probably anywhere else either. Polls showed that 90 percent of Americans knew about the Salk vaccine trials—more people than could have named the president of the United States. On April 12, 1955—the tenth anniversary of Franklin Roosevelt's death—at ten o'clock in the morning Thomas Francis announced to a mob of reporters and visiting dignitaries that the Salk vaccine was safe and effective.

The story made headlines across the nation, and Jonas Salk became an instant hero. He and his family had gone to Michigan for the announcement and were stunned by the press uproar, the endless interviews, and the photography sessions. When they got back to Pittsburgh, Salk's five-year-old son Jonathan called a friend and said, "Hi, Billy, I'm back from my vacation, I'm famous and so is my Dad." How much it all mattered to Americans is suggested by Ardean Martin, who had been chairwoman for the Mothers' March on Polio for San Diego County. In April 1955 she went to nearby Lindbergh Field to pick up the first shipment of Salk vaccine for her area. "And I stood there with tears running down my cheeks and I just said, 'Thank you, God. Thank you.'"

But the next year there were problems. Of the millions of people who got the vaccine that year, 204 contracted polio, 50 were paralyzed, and 11 of them died. Salk, O'Connor, and many others were distraught. What had gone wrong? Eventually the problem was traced to a batch of vaccine produced by a certain pharmaceutical lab where proper procedures had not been followed. The problem stopped, and by 1957 the incidence of polio in the United States was down by 80 percent.

By 1959 Albert Sabin had his attenuated vaccine ready. It had

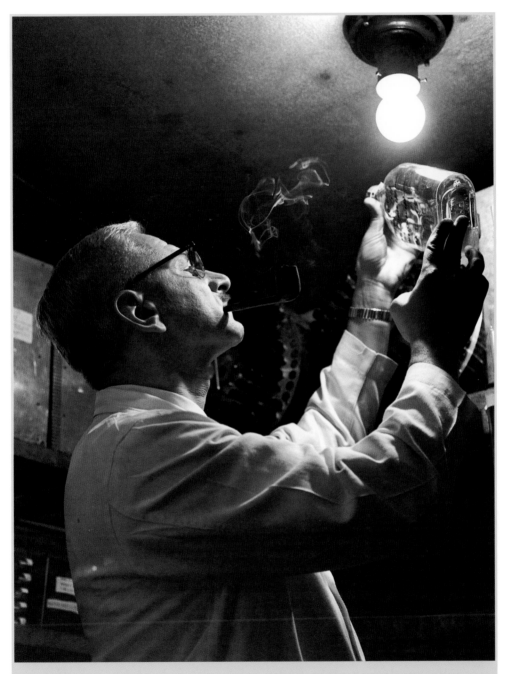

ALBERT SABIN DEVELOPED THE VACCINE GENERALLY FAVORED TODAY. IT CAN BE SWALLOWED IN ONE DOSE, WHEREAS THE SALK VACCINE REQUIRED THREE INJECTIONS.

considerable advantages over the Salk vaccine. Principally, where the Salk vaccine required three successive shots, the Sabin vaccine could be taken once, orally. Ironically, because so many people in the United States were now immune to polio because of the Salk vaccine, Sabin needed another source of subjects. He soon got the Russians, with whom polio had become a problem, to agree to tests. This was during the days of the Cold War, when the United States and the Soviet Union were bristling at each other and the possibility of war between the two countries seemed real. But in this case there was cooperation. In two years 77 million Russians got the Sabin vaccine, which proved a resounding success.

In 1961 the American Medical Association endorsed the Sabin vaccine, and within a few years it became the preferred one. It is today more widely used than the Salk vaccine. However the World Health Organization recommends the use of both. The incidence of polio in the United States is now down to about ten cases a year, which are mostly fluke results of the vaccine itself. The last case of polio from a natural virus in the Western Hemisphere occurred in Peru in 1991.

But polio is by no means dead elsewhere. It is endemic in sub-Sahara Africa, Central and South America, the eastern Mediterranean, and other places. There have been polio epidemics recently in Sudan (1993), Pakistan and Zaire (1995), and Albania (1996). Efforts today are being made to end the threat of polio worldwide by the World Health Organization and Rotary International, a private organization, and there is hope of eventual success.

There is, however, an unhappy postscript to the story. It has recently been discovered that people who suffered from polio in the past may get a second attack of the disease later in life. This "postpolio syndrome" may appear as many as fifty years after the first attack. Victims of postpolio syndrome often feel weak and tired, and may suffer from some muscles wasting away. It now seems that half of those who originally had the disease may be affected by postpolio syndrome. That is a lot of people; in the United States today there are some 600,000 polio survivors.

But presumably with the end of polio, there will in time be no more postpolio syndrome either. The fight against polio is one of the great medical success stories, like the conquest of smallpox. Polio was beaten in an astonishingly short time—less than forty years from the 1916 epidemic that first alerted the world to the disease until the introduction of the Salk vaccine. That is an amazing accomplishment.

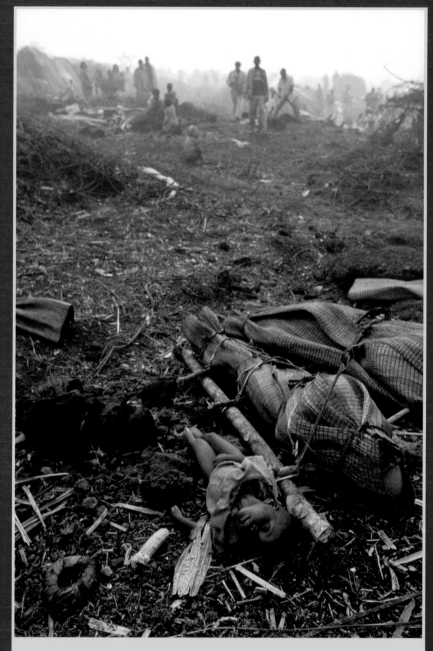

TODAY INFECTIOUS DISEASES RUN RAMPANT IN MANY DEVELOPING NATIONS. IN 1994 THOUSANDS OF RWANDAN REFUGEES FLEEING FIGHTING IN THEIR HOMELAND DIED FROM CHOLERA. THEIR BODIES WERE PILED BY THE SIDE OF THE ROAD NEAR A REFUGEE CAMP.

The Future

Today in the United States children routinely get—or are supposed to get—a series of vaccines. One of these is the so-called MMR vaccine, which protects against measles, mumps, and rubella (formerly called German measles). These were diseases that the parents of today's students took for granted as a part of their childhood; indeed, kids suffering from mumps were usually allowed all the ice cream they wanted, because it was less painful to swallow than other foods. Most American children now will never experience these diseases.

Polio and diphtheria vaccines are also routinely given. So is the vaccine for whooping cough (pertussis). In the past, children often suffered from whooping cough, which was not very dangerous if the case was mild, but could be debilitating in severe cases. We also vaccinate against type B influenza and since 1990 against meningitis, an inflammation of the brain and spinal cord. The vaccine has reduced the number of cases from 20,000 a year to 125. A vaccine for hepatitis B is standard in the United States, but not everywhere in the Western world. The disease can cause chronic liver damage and even death and affects tens of millions worldwide. Finally, Americans usually get a tetanus shot as children, but the vaccine is effective for only ten years, which is why people are given a tetanus booster shot when they get a puncture wound or an animal bite.

Unfortunately in the United States, a great many children today fall through the cracks. This country still does not offer a universal medical-insurance system that covers everybody. As a result the poor—especially immigrants who do not speak English well—are not given the first-class medical care that most Americans expect. Such children may not get all the shots they should. Not only are they subject to childhood diseases for which there are vaccines, but if they get sick they can expose others to them. One task for America today is to find ways to see that all children get the necessary vaccines.

Still, even these children get some protection. One of the advantages of breast-feeding infants is that they seem to get some natural immunity to some diseases in the process, although it may be temporary. Some of the mother's antibodies are passed along to the child through breast-feeding. Also, breast-fed babies seem to produce more antibodies in response to vaccines when they get them.

Exercise also seems to help develop the immune system. Some regular exposure to the sun is also good, although we are always warned not to overdo sun exposure because of the long-term risk of skin cancer.

After some 200 years, we no longer routinely give children the famous smallpox vaccine. The reason is simple: smallpox is no longer a threat to human beings. In 1967 the World Health Organization decided that it was possible to eradicate smallpox altogether. No infectious disease had ever been deliberately wiped out by human beings, and many people scoffed. But those who wanted to try pointed out that the smallpox virus did not mutate as readily as did some other microbes. There was no animal reservoir from which it could suddenly spring, as the Hong Kong flu had done. And one bout of smallpox gave protection for life. The disease had already been eliminated in most of the industrial nations, such as the United States and Japan; why not try to get rid of it in the developing nations where it still existed?

In one sense the task was easy: give everybody who might be in danger of smallpox a shot of the vaccine, and in time the virus would be wiped out. The problem was logistical: how do you track down all the susceptible people? And once having tracked them down, how do you persuade tribal people living in savannas and rain forests, with no understanding of the germ theory of disease, much less the complexities of immunology, to get the necessary shot? The goal was tremendous. For ten years health workers went into the rain forests and savannas, explaining what they were doing in hundreds of languages and persuading people to have the shots. Sometimes they were helped by local leaders who became convinced. But in at least one case, when a local chief refused to let his people be vaccinated, frustrated workers simply tackled the man and held him down while he was given the shot. He then quickly allowed his people to be vaccinated. The result was that in October 1977 the last natural case of smallpox was reported in Somalia.

There has, however, been considerable controversy about a few remaining samples of the frozen smallpox virus, left over from lab work, remaining in the United States and Russia. Many people think this remaining smallpox virus should be destroyed to prevent it from somehow escaping into the human population. However, some think the samples ought to be preserved in case smallpox appears again and viruses are needed for experimentation. The United States and Russia have agreed to destroy these samples, but as each deadline approaches, the governments have been persuaded to postpone the destruction. No one is sure what will eventually happen.

What we can be sure of, however, is that there will be more new diseases coming along. In particular there is a group caused by what are called emerging viruses. Some of these diseases have made headlines; some have not. Well-known is the Marburg virus, which afflicted twenty-five workers in Marburg, Germany, and Belgrade, in what was then Yugoslavia. All the people had all been handling certain monkeys shipped to Europe for laboratory purposes. Seven of the people died.

Related to Marburg is the Ebola virus, which caused epidemics in Africa after its first appearance in 1976. The death rate from Ebola has

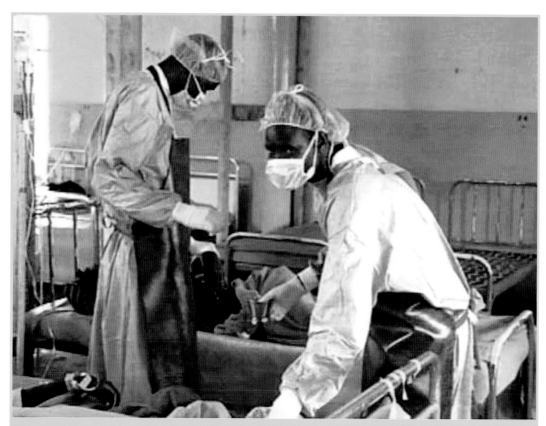

So far Ebola has been contained, but it has by no means been defeated. There is always the threat that it will be the source of a future full-scale epidemic. Here medical staff in Uganda try to save an Ebola victim in 2000.

been terrifying—up to 90 percent in some instances. Other emerging viruses include dengue fever, Rift Valley fever, Argentine hemorrhagic fever, and Japanese encephalitis. These are not all exotic diseases found only in foreign places: dengue fever has appeared in the United States.

More importantly the United States has in the past twenty years or so seen the establishment of two serious diseases that most Americans have heard about, and many have actually gotten. One of these is Lyme disease. In 1975 two mothers in the quaint Connecticut town of Old Lyme were upset by persistent illnesses in their children, which included fevers and aches in their joints. They discovered that other families had suffered from the same disease. Local doctors had diagnosed it as juvenile rheumatoid arthritis, but that particular disease had never before produced so many cases in one area. Several of the victims had noticed tick bites at the time the symptoms first appeared. Fortunately one of the victims had captured a tick from his skin and turned it over to a team at Yale University, located in nearby New Haven, Connecticut. Eventually the cause of Lyme disease was discovered: a bacterium carried by the so-called deer tick, a tiny animal about the size of the period at the end of this sentence. The deer tick goes through a complex life cycle during which it moves around among a variety of animals, especially rodents, and eventually lands in the grass, where it then may attach itself to a human. As it feeds on human blood, it passes the Lyme bacteria into the human system.

The number of cases of Lyme disease increased twenty times between 1982 and 1992, and has increased subsequently. It exists everywhere, but most cases have appeared in the Northeast, upper Midwest, and the West Coast. In northeastern states, such as New York and Connecticut, people who spend a lot of time outdoors, such as hunters and gardeners, are very likely to get Lyme disease. It is hard to diagnose, because the symptoms are not the same in everybody. If allowed to go untreated, it can cause serious problems such as arthritis, facial paralysis, and heart damage. Fortunately it can be treated with antibiotics, which usually stop the disease in a few days.

The second of the new microbial diseases we have heard much of in recent years is HIV, which causes AIDS. This disease is related to similar diseases in monkeys and may have spread from them to humans, but there is much debate about the origin of AIDS. It may have been in humans for some time, perhaps centuries. Then, with the boom in travel in the twentieth century triggered by supersonic planes, roads, and railroads able to reach formerly remote places, the disease began to spread.

Today it exists almost everywhere. It is spread by direct contact, usually sexual, or when the virus is actually injected into the bloodstream during a transfusion using infected blood, or by a drug user employing a dirty hypodermic needle.

There is no cure for AIDS, although new treatments have been worked out that prolong the life of the victim. The problem is that the AIDS virus attacks the immune system itself. In the end the victim usually dies from some disease that the weakened immune system can no longer fend off. AIDS has caused many deaths in the United States, but the deaths from AIDS in America are small compared with what is happening in Africa, where the disease has reached epidemic proportions in some areas. If a cure is not found soon, and it does not appear likely, AIDS will eventually kill tens of millions of Africans.

It should be clear to readers that animals are involved in a lot of these diseases, especially the emerging viruses that we have been looking at. Hong Kong flu came from chickens; certain species of mosquitoes carry dengue fever; Ebola and AIDS depend on monkey reservoirs; Lyme disease is stored in animal reservoirs. Particularly instructive is the example of Argentine hemorrhagic fever. It is carried by a species of mouse that flourished in the relatively empty grasslands of Argentina. After World War II, a lot of these grasslands were plowed in order to plant corn. The mice then spread into the cornfields and began infecting the farmworkers.

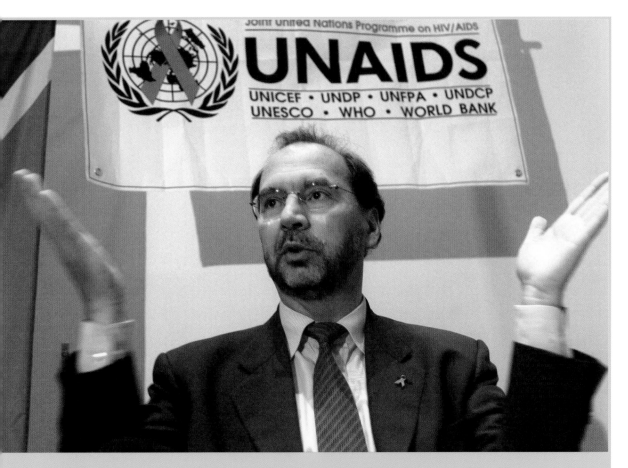

AIDS HAS ALREADY REACHED EPIDEMIC PROPORTIONS IN AFRICA AND CONTINUES TO KILL PEOPLE ALL
OVER THE WORLD. IN 2001 THE UNITED NATIONS, RESPONSIBLE FOR HELPING PREVENT THE SPREAD OF
AIDS, MARKED THE TWENTIETH ANNIVERSARY OF THE FIRST REPORTED CASES OF THE DISEASE. BY THEN IT
HAD KILLED 22 MILLION PEOPLE WORLDWIDE, AND RESEARCH INDICATES THAT THE EPIDEMIC IS ONLY IN ITS
EARLY STAGES.

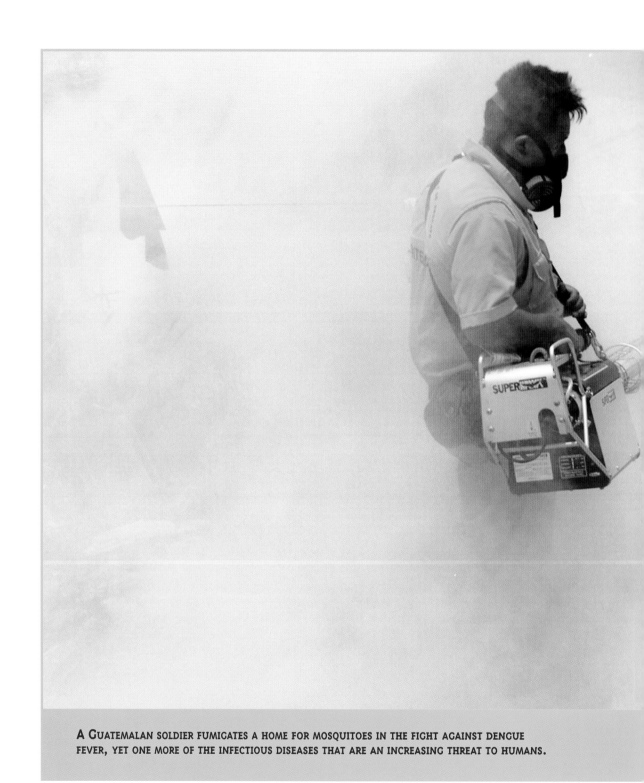

A Guatemalan soldier fumigates a home for mosquitoes in the fight against dengue fever, yet one more of the infectious diseases that are an increasing threat to humans.

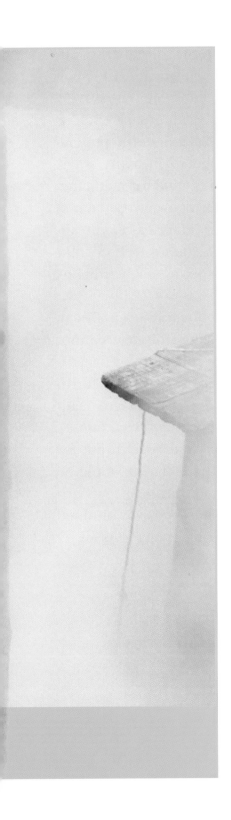

We can, of course, hope that scientists will come up with new vaccines for the diseases that afflict so many tens of millions of humans today. But more than vaccines are needed. Consider, for example, the case of polio. It became a serious problem in the United States because of social and political factors—principally unsanitary cities. It was ended also because of political and social factors—the great fear, especially in parents, that drove tens of thousands of them to volunteer in various polio campaigns; the prosperity of the United States which permitted Americans to raise the millions of dollars needed for research and the distribution of the vaccine; the fact that a very popular president had suffered from the disease and acted as a focus for the polio campaign; and perhaps most important, the fact that the United States was a society with good transportation, communication, and a vast array of medical institutions consisting of hospitals, schools, and research centers.

Few of these things exist in large numbers in many African nations, or in many other parts of the developing world, such as Cambodia and Myanmar in Southeast Asia, nations in the Middle East, and elsewhere. Particularly since the end of World War II, these places have been struggling to join the industrialized world, but with only partial success.

As a consequence, with the best will in the world it is frequently difficult for international groups to bring good medical practices to such countries. For example, the polio vaccine is available, it is relatively cheap, and the World Health Organization and private groups such as Rotary International are making strong efforts to vaccinate the populations of developing countries. But they are hampered in many ways. Lack of education leaves many people mistrustful of modern medicine. The chaos of rapidly expanding cities, often suffering from the lack of sanitation that was typical of nineteenth-century America, is yet another problem. Then there are deadly curiosities, such as the current African leader who continues to insist that there is no such thing as AIDS.

In the end, disease is not merely a medical problem: it is a political, social, and economic one as well. The battle against disease cannot truly be mounted until some of these problems are solved.

Living in the United States at this time, we are exceedingly fortunate, because we have been the primary benefactors of the great advances made in fighting infectious diseases in the past 200 years or so. Look around at your classmates sometime: if this had been 1850, for example, probably a third of them would not be there. There would be among them one or two crippled students wearing braces, a few with their faces scarred by smallpox, and others with their eyesight dimmed by disease. Vaccines have truly been a magnificent blessing for us all.

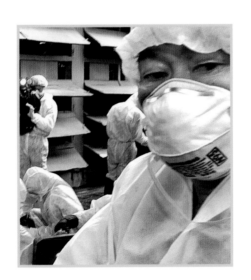

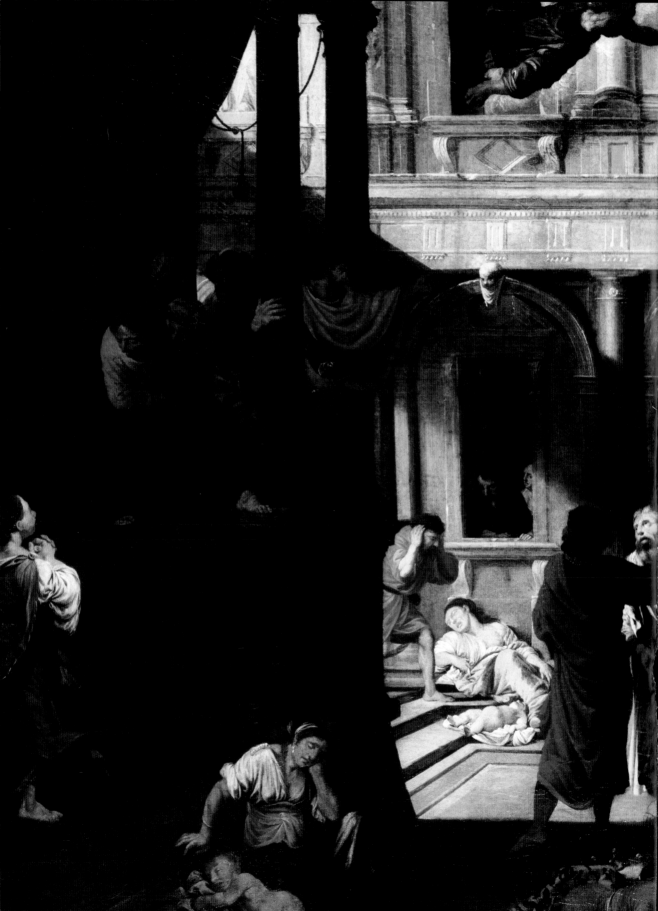

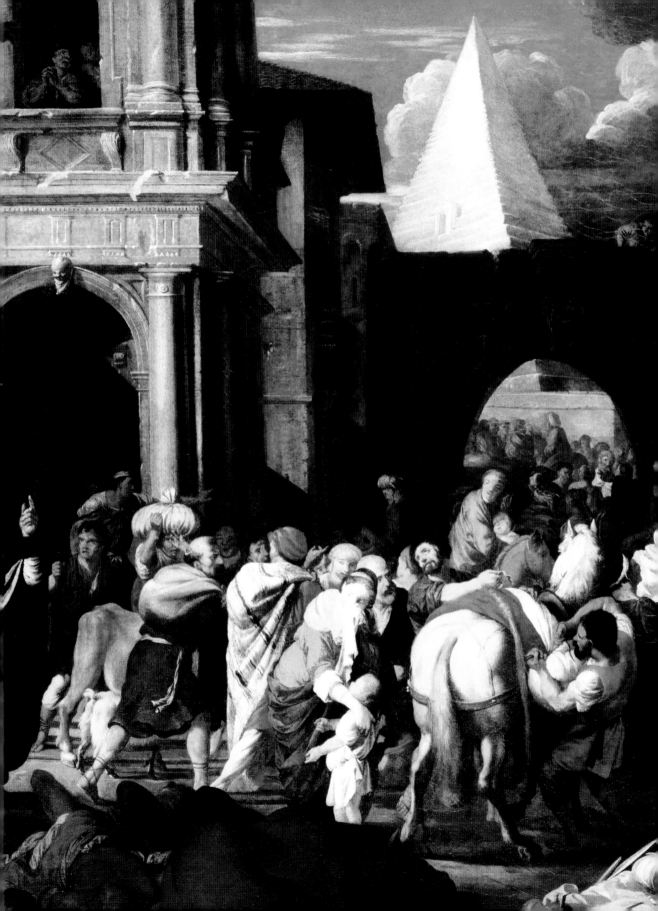

History of the Black Death
http://www.bbc.co.uk/history/society_culture/welfare/blackdeath/black_22.shtml

The Black Death, 1348
http://www.ibiscom.com/plague.htm

Plague's Effect on European Civilization
http://www.insecta-inspecta.com/fleas/bdeath/Europe.html

Louis Pasteur Links
http://inventors.about.com/library/inventors/blpasteur.htm

History and Achievements of Vaccines
http://www.immunizationinfo.org/parents/vaccineHistory.cfm

Bibliography

Books

FOR STUDENTS

Gosling, Peter J. *Pasteur: A Beginner's Guide*. London: Hodder and Stoughton, 2001.

Karlen, Arno. *Biography of a Germ*. New York: Anchor, 2001.

Peters, C. J., and Mark Olshaker. *Virus Hunter*. New York: Anchor, 1997.

Zinsser, Häns. *Rats, Lice and History*. New York: Bantam, 1965.

FOR TEACHERS

Debré, Patrice. *Louis Pasteur*. Baltimore: Johns Hopkins University Press, 1994.

Karlen, Arno. *Man and Microbes*. New York: Simon and Schuster, 1995.

McNeill, William H. *Plagues and People*. New York: Anchor, 1977.

Index

Page numbers for illustrations are in **boldface**.

Africa. *See* developing nations
AIDS, 89, 110, **111**
air quality, 25
animal reservoirs, 19–20, **85**, 85–86, 106, 110
anthrax, 57–59, 66
antibodies, 74–75, 81, 106
antitoxin, 73
Argentine hemorrhagic fever, 109, 110
art, 22, **24**
Athens, 22
Aztecs, **28**, 29

bacteria, 45–46, 49–51, 53–56, 65–66
    cultures, 65–66
    staining, 66
    weakening, 49, 56, 57–58
Behring, Emil, 73
Black Death. *See* bubonic plague
bloodletting, 33
boosters, 105
breast feeding, 106

bubonic plague, 11–22, **14–15**, 29, **47**

cancer, 25, 106
Center for Disease Control (CDC), 85
childbirth, 54–55
childhood, death in, 9–10
cholera, 70–72, 89, **104**
    in chickens, 56
cities, 10–11, **12–13**, 14, 16, 19, 46,
    66–69, **67**, **68**, 70, 71, 72, 89–90,
    114
contagion, 30, 46
costumes, **47**
cowpox, 34–38, **36–37**, **40–41**
cultural factors, 113–114
culture
    of bacteria, 65–66
    of influenza virus, 83

decaying matter, 45–46, 48–49, 51, 55
definitions, 30

dengue fever, 109, 110, **112–113**

developing nations, **104**, 106–107, 110, **111**, 113–114

diphtheria, 72–73, **73**, 105

disease
> causes, 16, **17**, 18, 30–31, **44**, 45–48, 53–56, 66
> effects, 22–23, 102–103, 114
> endemic, 30
> noninfectious, 25
> spread of, 30, 46–48, **47**, **52–53**, 66–69, **67**, **68**, 70, 96
> strains of, 37–38, 75, 83–85, 87, 97

doctors, **17**, 18, **52–53**, 54–55

Ebola virus, 107–109, **108**, 110

electron microscopes, 80, **80**, 83–84

encephalitis, 109

environmental causes, 25

epidemics, 22, 25–26, 70–71, 85–87, 90–92, 107–109, 110
> definition, 30
> *See also* bubonic plague; pandemics

ethics, 38

exercise, 106

experiments. *See* human trials

fermentation, 48–51

filters, 59

fleas, 19–21

flies and maggots, 45–46, 48–49

genes, 25

germ theory, 53–56, 66

heat, 49, 57–58

hemophilus influenza, 89

hepatitis B, 105

Hong Kong flu, **85**, 85–86

hospitals, **52–53**, 54–55

human trials
> by Jenner, 38–42, **39**
> by Pasteur, 51, 58, 62
> of Sabin vaccine, 102
> of Salk vaccine, 98–100

hydrophobia, 59

immune system, 73–75, 81, 106, 110

immunity, 27–29, 30, 56, 81, 106

Industrial Revolution, 66–69, **67**, **68**

inflammation, 74

influenza, 25–26, 75, **76**, **79**, 81–86, **86**, 105
> drugs against, 87
> hemophilus, 89
> from Hong Kong, **85**, 85–86
> in pigs, 83, 84

inoculation, **8**, 31–33, 34, **39**, 56, **60**
> definition, 30
> *See also* Jenner, Edward; vaccines

Japanese encephalitis, 109

Jenner, Edward, 33–43, **35**, **36–37**, **39**, **40–41**, 48

Koch, Robert, 57, **64**, 65–66, 69–70, 72

Leeuwenhoek, Antonie van, 45, 49
life expectancy, 9–10
Lister, Joseph, **54**, 55
Little Ice Age, 11
Lyme disease, 109–110
lymphocytes, 74–75

Marburg virus, 107
March of Dimes, 93–96, **94**, 98–99
measles, 29, 105
medicines, 87
Meister, Joseph, 62–63
meningitis, 105
miasma theory, 46–48, 66, 69, 72
microscopes, 45, 51, 66
    electron, 80, **80**, 83–84
Middle Ages, 10–11, 21–22, **44**
    See also bubonic plague
monkeys, 110
Montagu, Mary W., 31–32
morality, 18
mosquitoes, 110, **112–113**
mumps, 105

Native Americans, 27–30, **28**, 43
nutrition, 25

O'Connor, Basil, 93–96, 98–99
oxygen, 56, 58

pandemics, 30, 71, **76**, 77–79, 81–82
Pasteur, Louis, 48–53, **50**, **54**, 55–63, **60**,
    65, 72

pasteurization, 49
pathogens, 73
penitents, 19, **20**
pertussis, 105
pestilence, 14
Petri, Robert, 66
plague, 14
    See also bubonic plague
plug drugs, 87
polio, **88**, 89–103, **91**, 105, 113
prehistoric times, 30–31
prevention, 46, **47**, 49, 51, 54–55, **76**, **79**,
    112–113
    See also inoculation; sanitation
Progressives, 89–90
putrefaction, 45–46, 48–49, 51, 55

rabies, **57**, 59–62, **60**
rats, 19–21
religion, 16, 18–19, **20**, 29, 32, 43
resistance. *See* immunity
Rift Valley fever, 109
Roman Empire, **24**, 26–27
Roosevelt, Franklin D., 92–93, **93**
Roux, Emile, 73
rubella, 105

Sabin, Albert, 97–98, 99, 100–102, **101**
Salk, Jonas, 97, **98**, 98–99
sanitation, **52–53**, 54–55, 66–69, **67**, **68**,
    70, 71, 72, 89–90, 96, 114
satire, **40–41**
scurvy, 25

seasons, 14

Semmelweis, Ignaz, 54

ships, 21, 25, 46, 48

Shope, Richard E., 82–83

silkworm disease, 51–53

skin, 74, 106

smallpox, 23, 26–33, 43, 106–107
    See also Jenner, Edward

smog, 25

smoking, 25

Snow, John, 71

spitting, 70

spontaneous generation, 45–46, 48–49, 51

starvation, 33

sterilization, 54–55

Stone Age, 30–31

strains, of disease, 37–38, 75, 83–85, 87, 97

sun, 106

surgery, 54–55

swine flu, 83, 84

temperaments, **44**

tetanus, 105

ticks, 109

Toussaint, J. J. H., 57

travel, 11–14, **12–13**, 21, 48, 70–71, 78,
    87, 110

tuberculosis, 69–70, **74**, 89

typhoid fever, **8**

United States, **8**, 30, 43, 71, 78, 85,
    105–106, 109–110
    See also cities; influenza; polio

vaccines
    for anthrax, 57–59
    for cholera, 56
    etymology, 42
    and immunity, 75
    for influenza, 84–85, 87, 105
    manufacture of, 100
    measles, mumps, rubella (MMR), 105
    for polio, 89, 96
    for rabies, 61–62
    routine U. S., 105–106
    for smallpox, 106–107 (*see also*
    smallpox)
    for tuberculosis, 69–70

viruses, 59–61, 79–81, 84, 107–109, **108**
    See also AIDS; influenza; polio;
    smallpox

vitamins, 25

water, 18, 69, 71–72

weather, 11

Web sites, 119

white blood cells, 74–75

whooping cough, 105

World War I, 78, 82

yeast, 49

zoonosis, 30

About the Author

James Lincoln Collier has written books for both adults and students on many subjects, among them the prizewinning novel *My Brother Sam Is Dead*. Many of these books, both fiction and nonfiction, have historical themes, including the highly acclaimed Benchmark Books series the Drama of American History, which he wrote with Christopher Collier.